NURS PROCESS

PROCESS

Concepts and Application

Second Edition

Wanda Walker Seaback, RN, BSN
Professor of Nursing
Kingwood College
Kingwood, Texas

THOMSON

DELMAR LEARNING™

Australia Canada Mexico Singapore Spain United Kingdom United States

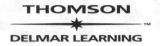

THOMSON

DELMAR LEARNING

Nursing Process: Concepts and Application, Second Edition
by Wanda Seaback

Vice President, Health Care Business Unit:
William Brottmiller

Editorial Director:
Cathy L. Esperti

Acquisitions Editor:
Melissa Martin

Editorial Assistant:
Tiffiny Adams

Marketing Director:
Jennifer McAvey

Marketing Channel Manager:
Tamara Caruso

Marketing Coordinator:
Michele Gleason

Production Director:
Carolyn Miller

Production Editor:
Jack Pendleton

Library of Congress Cataloging-in-Publication Data

Seaback, Wanda Walker.
  Nursing process : concepts and
    application / Wanda Walker
Seaback.–2nd ed.
  p. ; cm.
  ISBN-13 978-1-4018-1989-7
  ISBN-10 1-4018-1989-3
  1. Nursing–Problems, exercises, etc.
  2. Nursing–Examinations, questions, etc.
  [DNLM: 1. Nursing Process–Problems
and Exercises. WY 18.2 S438n 2006]
  I. Title.

  RT55.S42 2006
  610.73'076–dc22

                              2005012887

NOTICE TO THE READER

To Dr. Steve Sansom, North Harris College, Houston, TX. Professor, English:
Thank you for raising the bar a little higher, encouraging creativity and confidence in your students, and teaching more than the fundamentals of writing and expressing oneself.

To Orville Walker: Thanks Dad for always being there for me. Your example of how to live a faith-filled life has been a guiding influence in the lives of your children, grandchildren, and great-grandchildren. Your legacy will live on for many years to come.

Table of Contents

Preface

Nursing Process: Concepts and Application was written with the educator and nursing student in mind. Most educators will agree, the nursing process is one of the most important concepts to be taught in fundamental nursing. Most theories presented in nursing textbooks are based on the nursing process steps: assessment, problem identification/diagnosis, planning and outcome identification, implementation, and evaluation. National licensing examination questions are formatted and written utilizing the nursing process.

The student textbook is written to correspond with the educator's PowerPoint presentation/lecture material (included on the accompanying CD). Numerous learning activities and key points are included throughout each chapter, thus promoting interactive learning and stimulating student questions and in-class discussion. Activities are necessary for students to understand the presented concepts and theory and for practical application of these concepts. The student's textbook is written in a format designed to make learning fun. The author's goal was to maintain a clear, uncluttered approach emphasizing application.

The appendices include a complete current list of NANDA nursing diagnoses for easy reference. Once the textbook is completed, it becomes an important reference for the student to use throughout nursing education.

Key Features:
- The interactive student text and the educator presentations are linked so that the student can follow along, completing the text and interacting in the class discussion.
- Text presents the nursing process in an easy-to-understand, step-by-step format.
- Student Practice activities promote application of the concept behind each step.
- Student Practice activities build upon one another, increasing in complexity to promote understanding, critical thinking, and practical application of each step of the nursing process.
- Numerous examples and cases allow students to apply their knowledge as they progress through the text.

WHAT'S NEW IN THE SECOND EDITION?

Sample chapters of the first draft were selected and sent for review by nurse educators in colleges of nursing throughout the United States. Reviewers were faculty in licensed vocational/practical nursing programs, associate degree and baccalaureate programs. Those nursing professionals were asked specific questions, such as, what was liked about the sample, what was not liked, and what would improve the textbook. These comments were shared with the author and have been used to guide the revisions and additions in the second edition, which include the following:

- Additional theory and graphics have been included. Chapter 1 provides theoretical concepts and foundation information. Chapters 2 through 6 discuss each step of the nursing process, introducing key terms, examples, points to remember, and learning activities. Chapter 7 helps the student put it all together. A clinical case study is presented and the author takes the student through each step.

The final product is a documented care plan representative of the clinical responses one client may exhibit resulting from his condition.

- The fill-in-the-blank copy has been eliminated, so that students may prepare for lecture by reading material prior to class.
- Expanded case studies and additional examples are provided throughout each chapter.
- Improved PowerPoint material is included on the accompanying CD for the educator, as well as possible answers to student activities and case studies.
- Each chapter builds upon the next. Activities are provided to reinforce material learned.
- Activities are conducive to individual or group participation.

THE AUTHOR'S CONCEPT

In developing this textbook, I desired a work that could be adapted to all levels of nursing education, beginning with vocational/practical, applied science/associate degree nursing, and then broadening concepts and theory to embrace baccalaureate nursing. I believed it was important to present essential material students must learn and understand in order to apply the nursing process in clinical practice.

I was motivated to compose an instruction manual with an accompanying student workbook, providing important basic information and laying a foundation, step-by-step, that each student could understand and apply. Since its initial development in 1996, a great deal of the content has been rewritten and revised for clarity and effectiveness to benefit students' understanding. I was pleased to find that my nursing students, through the use of this text, were finally able to understand the concepts and demonstrated the ability to apply their knowledge to clinical practice. My students consistently demonstrate an overall improvement in critical thinking and clinical application through the use of this text. *Nursing Process: Concepts and Application* is the culmination of this endeavor.

The author invites students and nursing professors to send comments or recommendations via e-mail. Many of your observations and annotations have been influential in the revisions of this manuscript. E-mail: **wseaback@nhmccd.edu**

Nursing Process and Providing Care

"... observation and experience will teach us the ways to maintain or to bring back the state of health."

Florence Nightingale

OBJECTIVES

Upon completion of this chapter, the student should be able to:

- Describe the historical evolution of the nursing process.
- Discuss the nursing process as a therapeutic framework and describe how it is accepted as a tool for promoting multidisciplinary collaboration.
- List and define the five steps of the nursing process.
- Identify theories and philosophies nursing professionals use in practice to gain an understanding of the human race.
- Explain how critical thinking is an important element of the nursing process.
- List outstanding characteristics and benefits of the nursing process.

KEY TERMS

actual nursing diagnosis
assessment
care plan
client centered
collaboration
collaborative problem
critical thinking
decision making
diagnosis

evaluation
expected outcome
goal
implementation
JCAHO
medical diagnosis
NANDA
nursing diagnosis
nursing intervention

nursing process
objective data
prioritize
problem solving
process
risk nursing diagnosis
strengths
subjective data
wellness nursing diagnosis

The nursing process is a step-by-step method of providing care to clients. While progressing through each step, the nurse uses a variety of skills that are purposeful and promote a systematic, orderly thought process. The nursing process consists of five steps—assessment, diagnosis, planning and outcome identification, implementation, and evaluation.

This chapter provides a brief historical time line of the evolution of the nursing process (see Table 1:1), its outstanding characteristics, and an overview of each step. Chapter topics include discussion of the theoretical basis of the nursing process, the importance and necessity of critical thinking throughout all steps of the process, and the relationship between problem solving, decision making, and the nursing process.

John T., a Registered Nurse (RN), receives a shift report less than an hour ago on his assigned group of patients. As he organizes his notes, preparing for the day, the nursing assistant reports an extremely elevated blood pressure (210/108) for Mrs. Simpson in room 214-B.

Clinical situations, such as the scenario above, are likely to occur in most health care institutions. If you are the nurse, what will you do next? What is the priority for care? What questions will you ask? What actions will you take?

Understanding and applying concepts of the nursing process will help the nurse identify priorities, plan, provide health care, and evaluate patient progress. What is the *nursing process*?

Read on for the definition of the nursing process and examples of application!

WHAT IS A PROCESS?

The term process is defined as a series of planned actions or operations directed toward a particular result or goal.

NURSING PROCESS

The nursing process is defined as an organized, systematic method of planning and providing individualized care to clients. The nursing process is a tool promoting organization and utilization of the steps to achieve desired outcomes. The steps of the nursing process build upon each other, overlapping previous and subsequent steps. The nursing process may be used with clients throughout their life span and in any setting where care is provided to clients.

TABLE 1:1 Timeline: Evolution of the Nursing Process

pre-1955	Before the nursing process evolved, the nurse provided care based on medical orders written by physicians. Care was initiated based on the caregiver's instinct to nurture. There were no clearly identifiable boundaries defined for nursing practice.
1955	The term nursing process was coined by Lydia Hall.
Late 1950's– early 1960's	Dorothy Johnson (1959), Ida Orlando (1961), and Ernestine Wiedenbach (1963) introduced a three-step nursing process model.
1966	Virginia Henderson identified the nursing process model as the same steps used in the scientific method: observing, measuring, gathering data, and analyzing the findings.
1967	A four-step model was proposed: assessment, planning, intervention, and evaluation.
1973	The use of the nursing process in clinical practice continued to gain additional accuracy and recognition when the American Nurses Association (ANA) published *Standards of Clinical Nursing Practice* (Table 1:2).
	Publication of Standards gave further legitimacy to the five phases or steps of the nursing process. Nursing educators and clinicians began to use the five-step nursing process model on a regular basis. National conferences were initiated in 1973, resulting in the beginning of the classification of nursing diagnoses. North American Nursing Diagnosis Association (NANDA) conferences have been held every two years since then for the purpose of identification, clarification, and refinement of nursing diagnoses.
1980	ANA published a social policy statement, which provided guidelines (standards) for individual professional nurses to follow in practice.
1982	National Council Licensure Examination (NCLEX) was revised to include the nursing process concepts as a basis for organization.
1984	Joint Commission on Accreditation of Health care Organizations (JCAHO) launched requirements for accredited hospitals to use the nursing process as a means of documenting all phases of client care.
Current	The nursing process is a five-step process: assessment, diagnosis, planning, implementation, and evaluation.

TABLE 1:2 Scope and Standards of Practice

Standard 1	*Assessment* The registered nurse collects comprehensive data pertinent to the patient's health or the situation.
Standard 2	*Diagnosis* The registered nurse analyzes the assessment data to determine the diagnoses or issues.
Standard 3	*Outcomes Identification* The registered nurse identifies expected outcomes for a plan individualized to the patient or the situation.
Standard 4	*Planning* The registered nurse develops a plan that prescribes strategies and alternatives to attain expected outcomes.
Standard 5	*Implementation* The registered nurse implements the identified plan.
Standard 5A	*Coordination of Care* The registered nurse coordinates care delivery.
Standard 5B	*Health Teaching and Health Promotion* The registered nurse employs strategies to promote health and a safe environment.
Standard 5C	*Consultation* The advanced practice registered nurse and the nursing role specialist provide consultation to influence the identified plan, enhance the abilities of others, and effect change.
Standard 5D	*Prescriptive Authority and Treatment* The advanced practice registered nurse uses prescriptive authority, procedures, referrals, treatments, and therapies in accordance with state and federal laws and regulations.
Standard 6	*Evaluation* The registered nurse evaluates progress toward attainment of outcomes.

From American Nurses Association (2004). *Nursing: Scope and standards of practice.* Washington, DC: Author.

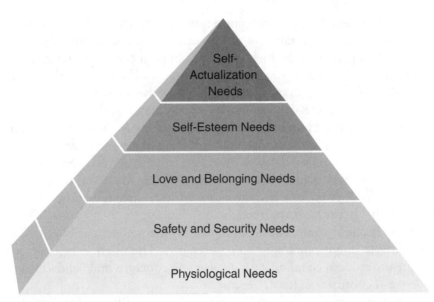

FIGURE 1:1 Maslow's Hierarchy of Needs. All human beings have common basic needs that must be met to some degree before higher-level needs are met.

Unique Characteristics of the Nursing Process

The nursing process is a problem-solving and decision-making method that is scientifically, as well as philosophically, based. The nurse uses learned knowledge and understanding of the human body to identify actual or potential health problems resulting from physical or psychological diseases or disorders. Knowledge and understanding of fundamental philosophical views, such as Maslow's hierarchy of human needs (Figure 1:1), are essential to the practice of nursing and aid in identifying the expected response to illness or the client's sense of wellness.

The nursing process is cyclic, ongoing, and dynamic. Using an orderly, step-by-step process, the client is evaluated, data are collected and analyzed, and a plan is formulated and set into motion. Client progress and response to treatment are continuously monitored and evaluated. The care plan is revised according to the changing needs of the client.

TABLE 1:3 Comparing Nursing and Nonnursing Models

Nursing Models	Nonnursing Models
• Functional health patterns • Human response pattern • Theory of self care	• Body systems model • Hierarchy of needs

Assessment models provide a systematic method for organizing data. Both nursing and nonnursing models (e.g., medical, psychology) are utilized (see Table 1:3).

The nursing process is a method used to organize nursing activities. The ultimate goal is to promote and restore client wellness, or to maintain the client's present state of health or sense of wellness.

The nursing process is recognized to be highly effective in promoting quality of care. A client entering the health care continuum receives a thorough initial assessment. The needs of the client are identified. A care plan (documentation of the first, second, and third steps of the nursing process) is developed and communicated to other health care professionals, so care is coordinated and ongoing. The client is continuously monitored for changing needs, and the plan is evaluated for accuracy. Assessment and evaluation, which are constant, play a key role in realizing client needs, strengths, and response to treatment. Health care professionals review, revise, and validate the care plan, enhancing and promoting quality of care.

The nursing process serves as a guide, ensuring deliberate steps are taken which help avoid omissions and premature conclusions. It provides a framework for which nurses use knowledge and skill to express human caring and to help clients meet their needs.

The nursing process is **client centered**, meaning care is focused on the client. The nurse organizes the care plan according to client problems and/or strengths. The client is encouraged to be an active participant in the nursing process, communicating needs and concerns and validating collected data. This gives the client a sense of control over his or her care.

Through the nursing process, the nurse utilizes interpersonal, technical, and intellectual skills.

- Interpersonal skills include communicating, listening, conveying interest and compassion, and sharing knowledge and information. The use of interpersonal skills aids in promoting trust.
- Technical skills deal with operation of equipment and performance of procedures.
- Intellectual skills involve cognitive measures, such as, analyzing, problem solving, critical thinking, and making judgments.

The nursing process promotes **collaboration** (communication with other disciplines to solve problems). As the client enters the health care system, individual professional responsibilities of the health care providers begin. Ongoing assessment of the client and response to care are monitored and recorded as physician orders and nursing interventions are carried out. Nursing professionals communicate necessary data through means of verbal reports and written documentation. Collaboration with the physician, nursing professionals, and other disciplines is often necessary to coordinate care and promote health.

The nursing process is universally applicable. It is appropriate to institute and apply the nursing process with clients of any age. The nursing process may be incorporated at any point on the wellness-illness continuum in a variety of health-related settings including schools, hospitals, home health care facilities and clinics, and across specialties in hospital or acute care settings including intensive care, pediatrics, labor and delivery, medical surgical units, etc.

Use of the nursing process is beneficial to both the client and nurse. Examples of benefits include the following:

- Promotes improved quality and continuity of care
- Promotes and encourages client participation
- Delivery of care and problem solving are organized, continuous, and systematic
- Time and resources are utilized more efficiently
- Delivery of care meeting expectations of both the health care consumer and standards of the nursing profession
- Holds all nurses accountable and responsible for assessment, diagnosis, planning, implementation, and evaluation of client care

Each step of the nursing process is specific, in sequence, and interrelated.

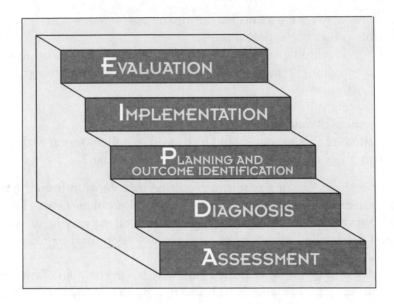

Step 1: Assessment

Assessment provides significant information, assembled to form the client database. This phase involves several steps:

1. Data collection: through interviews, conversations, and performing physical assessment. A variety of sources may be utilized for the purpose of data collection, i.e., the client, family, significant other, and review of diagnostic examinations, laboratory results, and the client's chart.
2. Verification: validating accuracy of data will help prevent omissions, misunderstanding, and incorrect inferences.
3. Organization: categorizing or identifying patterns in data
4. Interpretation: formulating initial ideas or impressions
5. Documentation: recording or reporting data

Two types of information are collected during the assessment step: objective and subjective data. Objective data are observable or measurable information, accumulated through the physical exam, interview, or results of diagnostic examinations. Subjective data include the client's communicated description, perception, feelings, emotions, or concerns. A more detailed description of objective and subjective data can be found in Chapter 2, "Assessment."

Step 2: Diagnosis

Diagnosis is the classification of a disease, condition, or human response based upon scientific evaluation of signs and symptoms, patient history, and diagnostic studies. Diagnosis involves analysis of collected data. After analysis, a list of nursing diagnoses or labels describing client problems or strengths is formulated. The nurse uses critical-thinking and decision-making skills in developing nursing diagnoses, a process facilitated by asking questions such as:

- What actual problems, if any, were identified during the assessment step?
- What are the possible causes of the problems?
- Is the client at risk for developing other problems; if so, what are the factors involved?
- Did the client indicate a desire to function at a higher level of wellness in a particular area?
- What are the client's strengths?
- What additional data might be needed to answer these questions?
- What are possible sources of data collection?
- Are there any identified problems that should be treated in collaboration with the physician?
- What data are pertinent to collect before contacting the physician?

During the diagnosis phase, existing problems requiring intervention from the nurse are identified. When the client demonstrates signs and symptoms, an actual problem exists. This type of problem is labeled as an **actual nursing diagnosis**. Potential problems a client may be at risk for developing are identified as well and are labeled as **risk nursing diagnoses**. Potential or risk problems may be prevented by actions executed for the purpose of prevention.

Wellness nursing diagnoses may be identified and included in the plan of care, when the client has indicated a desire to attain a higher level of wellness in a particular area. The diagnostic label is preceded by the phrase *potential for enhanced*. For example, a client who is neither overweight nor underweight expresses a desire to gain more knowledge on how to reduce overall fat content of her diet for future health and prevention of disease. The nurse would identify the wellness nursing diagnosis of *Potential for Enhanced Nutrition*.

Strengths of the client are identified. These are areas of positive functioning used to support the care plan. For example, a client's family may be very supportive, giving encouragement and the desire to get well.

Potential complications (PCs) requiring physician intervention that arise during treatment are identified and considered **collaborative problems**. Actions are initiated to resolve or reduce the risk of complication by implementing physician-prescribed orders in collaboration with nursing-prescribed interventions. The nurse primarily monitors for the onset and change in status of physiological complications. These usually are related to disease, trauma, treatments, medications, or diagnostic studies (Carpenito, 1997). Collaborative problems are labeled as *PC* followed by the situation, for example, a client who has undergone surgical intervention, *PC: Hemorrhage* or a client who has experienced a myocardial infarction, *PC: Dysrhythmias*.

Clients receive both medical and nursing diagnoses. *Nursing diagnoses* should not be confused with *medical diagnoses*. Table 1:4 compares medical and nursing diagnoses.

Medical diagnoses are determined by the physician or nurse practitioner indicating a disease or disorder identified or to be ruled out, e.g., pneumonia, renal failure, sepsis, or diabetes mellitus. Nursing diagnoses are problems identified and determined by the professional nurse. So, *what makes the nursing diagnosis different?*

According to the NANDA, a **nursing diagnosis** is a clinical judgment about individual, family, or community responses to actual or potential health problems/life processes. In 1980, the ANA defined nursing process as the diagnosis and treatment of human responses to actual or potential health problems of disease and medical treatment.

So, what's the difference?

MD:
"This client
has
pneumonia."

LPN:
"This client
is experiencing
Ineffective
Breathing
Pattern."

The preceding statement means nurses are *not* responsible for diagnosing and ordering treatment for disorders such as cancer. Professional nurses diagnose and treat the client's response to cancer, such as inadequate nutrition, nausea, altered self-esteem, anxiety, and pain.

After data are analyzed and problems, risks, and strengths identified, a list of nursing diagnoses is formulated, then presented to the client for confirmation. If the client is unable to participate, family members may be able to assist in confirmation. Finally, the list of nursing diagnoses is recorded and the remainder of the client's care plan completed.

TABLE 1:4 Comparison of Medical Diagnoses and Nursing Diagnoses

Medical Diagnoses	Nursing Diagnoses
• Determined by the provider • Indicate a disease or disorder identified or to be ruled out • Remain constant until client recovers from disease or illness	• Determined by nurses • Indicate the client's response to illness, disease, or present state of health • May change as the client responds to medical treatment, therapies, and nursing interventions
Examples: • Pneumonia • COPD exacerbation • Prostatitis • Acute renal failure	**Examples:** • Impaired gas exchange • Ineffective breathing pattern • Altered urinary elimination • Risk for impaired skin integrity

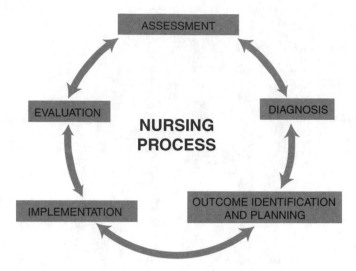

FIGURE 1:2 Nursing process is a method used to determine client needs. Assessment of the client and evaluation of the client and care plan are continuous. The nurse uses critical thinking, problem solving, and decision making throughout this process.

The client is continuously reassessed (Figure 1:2). Data are collected and documented during this process. As physician-prescribed treatments and nursing-prescribed interventions are carried out, the client demonstrates responses to the care provided. Response to treatment may involve improvement of health or the client's condition may worsen. Nursing diagnoses included in the care plan reflect the changing needs of the client.

Step 3: Planning and Outcome Identification

Planning and outcome identification involve formulating and documenting the care plan. This phase of the nursing process organizes the proposed course of action for resolution of actual problems and prevention of risk problems. This task involves several steps:

1. Prioritizing nursing diagnoses
2. Identifying short- and long-term goals and expected outcomes
3. Determining nursing interventions that will aid in resolution or prevention of each problem

Prioritizing problems means to decide which nursing diagnoses are most important and require attention first. Problems involving life-threatening situations are given the highest priority. An in-depth discussion of prioritizing problems can be found in Chapter 4.

The absolute goal for any client is to achieve or maintain the greatest level of wellness possible. Goals are client centered, which means they focus on *behavior* of the client. Goals are broad statements describing the intended or desired change in the client's condition. An expected outcome is a particular expectation involving steps leading to the fulfillment of a goal, and therefore, resolution of the cause of a problem. Goals and expected outcomes are used to evaluate the effectiveness of nursing interventions and the care plan.

Nursing interventions are activities executed to enable accomplishment of goals. They are nursing actions planned and implemented with problem resolution in mind.

Step 4: Implementation

Implementation involves execution of the nursing care plan. As planned interventions are performed, the nurse must continue to assess the client's condition before, during, and after each intervention is carried out. Reporting and documentation of collected data are important. Both positive and negative responses are reported and documented. Negative responses to treatment may require additional intervention. Chapter 5 provides an in-depth discussion of implementation. Implementation includes:

1. Activating the plan of care
2. Carrying out planned interventions
3. Continued assessment as interventions are carried out
4. Recording and documenting care provided, interventions carried out, and client responses

Step 5: Evaluation

During **evaluation** (appraisal of results), the nurse determines if client goals were met, partially met, or not met. If the goal has been met, the nurse must decide if or when nursing activities will cease. This decision will depend on the client's status. Can the client maintain the present level of wellness? If the goal has been partially met or not met, the nurse reactivates each step of the nursing process. Data must be collected to determine why the goal was not achieved and what modifications to the care plan are necessary. Refer to Table 1:5 for sample questions nurses ask to evaluate client care.

COGNITIVE SKILLS

When a client enters the health care system, nurses are involved in decision making. Care is planned for the client based on facts continuously collected and analyzed throughout the nursing process. Skills vital to this process include critical thinking, problem solving, and decision making.

TABLE 1:5 Questions to Ask During Evaluation

- Are the interventions working?
- Is the current care plan helping the client make progress toward the goal?
- Has the client's status changed in any way? If so, is the plan still valid?
- Was the goal met or partially met?
- Was the goal realistic?
- Is there more that the health care team can do?
- Was the time frame too optimistic?
- Are goals and nursing interventions appropriate for the client?

Critical Thinking

Critical thinking is a purposeful thought process incorporating various strategies in search for the meaning of data. Deliberate questions are asked in order to validate and evaluate evidence. Critical thinkers seek out explanations for what is happening. Examples of questions critical thinkers ask are found in Table 1:6.

Problem Solving

The nursing process is a problem-solving method. However, there is a difference between this method and the method used in solving daily problems. In both methods, information is gathered, problems are identified, specific problems are labeled, a plan is developed for solving the problem, the plan is put

TABLE 1:6 Questions Critical Thinkers May Ask

Assessment	Have any data been omitted? Are there any data to be verified or validated that otherwise would lead to possible inaccuracies? Do subjective data complement and clarify objective data?
Diagnosis	What meaning is attached to collected data? What else could this mean? When clustering data, is there a pattern indicating specific problems? Is the client demonstrating signs or symptoms indicating they are at risk of developing future problems? Do the nursing diagnosis label and etiology accurately describe the problem? Did the client have adequate input into problem identification?
Planning and Outcome Identification	What are priority problems? Why are these problems priorities? What are the goals for the client? Are these goals realistic? What else might be accomplished? What interventions can assist the client in goal attainment? Is collaboration with other medical or health-related sources beneficial at this time? What other resources could benefit the client? Are planned interventions appropriate for the client, nurse, and facility?
Implementation	Has the client's condition changed since the last interaction? What is the client's current status? What interventions should be carried out first? Is the client demonstrating improvement in health status? Did the executed intervention result in the expected response? Why did the client respond in that manner?
Evaluation	Is the client progressing toward goal attainment? Are goals being met or only partially met? Is there more that can be done to alter the situation? Can the care plan be revised to be more effective? Was information accurate when initial data were collected? Was assessment thorough? Was each additional step of the nursing process followed through appropriately? Should additional data be collected? How can the plan be revised to best suit the client's needs?

Nursing Tip

Think about the whole clinical picture.

If someone is having difficulty breathing or is in extreme pain . . .

Attend to this priority first!

into action, and then, the results are evaluated. However, in solving daily problems, plans are frequently based on incomplete data and sometimes on presumptions. This type of problem solving is more linear compared with the cyclic and ongoing nature of the nursing process. Nurses using the nursing process method of problem solving actively engage in taking deliberate steps and use critical thought to identify and solve problems.

Decision Making

Decision making, a skill used throughout the nursing process, is based on systematic and scientifically based theories. Appropriate decision making and problem solving result from the nurse's ability to think critically, using perceptual and intellectual skills. This results in accurate problem identification, generating a reflective care plan and determining appropriate nursing interventions to aid in problem resolution. Interventions for each nursing diagnosis are selected based on scientific rationale, *why* the intervention will work. An in-depth discussion of scientific rationales can be found in Chapter 4, "Planning."

KEY CONCEPTS

- The nursing process is an organized, continuous, systematic method of planning, providing care, and problem solving. It is cyclic, ongoing, and dynamic.
- When a client enters the health care system, the nursing process begins. Use of the nursing process improves quality of care provided and promotes continuity of care.
- The nursing process consists of five interrelated steps: assessment, diagnosis, planning and outcome identification, implementation, and evaluation.
- Data collection utilizes a variety of sources and tools (*assessment*). Efforts are instituted to prevent omission or collection of inaccurate data.
- Data are organized and analyzed. Problems, potential problems, and strengths are identified and labeled (*diagnosis*).
- During the planning and outcome identification step, nursing diagnoses are prioritized. The professional nurse makes decisions on an appropriate course of action. The plan focuses on the client.
- Interventions are carried out (*implementation*).

- *Evaluation* of the plan and reassessment of the client are ongoing and continuous. The care plan is revised and updated when the client's needs change in response to medical treatment, therapies, and nursing interventions.
- *Care plan* revision may be necessary when the goal of treatment is partially met or not met.
- The care plan is developed, recorded, and placed in the client's chart, then communicated to other health care team members. This promotes ongoing continuity of care. The plan is reviewed for accuracy according to the policy of the facility and revised when needed.
- Nurses use perceptual and intellectual skills such as critical thinking, problem solving, and decision making.

APPLICATION EXAMPLE 1: PROBLEM SOLVING

Rachel Hernandez, a nurse for several years, was getting ready for a busy week. She was to drop her daughter, Marie, off at school before reporting for her shift at the local hospital. Marie had not responded when she was called for breakfast.

Step 1: Assessment

Ms. Hernandez was concerned and began to investigate the situation. As she approached Marie, her face looked flushed and she complained of fatigue. When she got closer, she could see red, raised, rashes all over her face and arms. Marie began scratching and reported she itched. Ms. Hernandez assessed for additional signs and symptoms. Marie's oral temperature was 98.8°F and the glands in her neck were slightly swollen. Numerous questions went through Ms. Hernandez's mind as she performed a physical assessment and asked important questions. Marie was adamant she was not going to school looking like this!

Step 2: Diagnosis

Ms. Hernandez was unsure of Marie's medical diagnosis; however, she was able to identify two distinct problematic responses resulting from her condition. The responses were labeled using approved NANDA nursing diagnoses:

Impaired Skin Integrity. Related to (RT): presence of unknown infectious process; as evidenced by (AEB): pruritus, erythematous (red), raised rash on face and arms.

Step 3: Planning

- Ms. Hernandez thought about the preceding problems and what could be done. During the planning phase, questions are asked relating to problem solving. Is collaboration with other experts necessary or warranted? What independent activities can be done that are within my scope of practice and knowledge? What outcome can and should be achieved? What steps should be taken to resolve the situation?
- For impaired skin integrity, the primary goal/outcome is for Marie to demonstrate evidence of timely healing of the skin lesions, without complications and within a reasonable amount of time, such as, over the next 72 hours.
- Next in planning is to develop a plan of action and determine priorities.

  1. Contact Marie's school to report she would be absent for the day.
  2. Contact the family physician for an afternoon appointment.

3. Stress not to scratch the lesions and to keep the area clean/dry.
4. Provide instructions for taking Tylenol for an elevated temperature if needed.

Step 4: Implementation

• Continue to assess Marie as interventions are executed. Carry out and perform the planned interventions.

Step 5: Evaluation

• Evaluation involves asking questions such as: Did the plan work? Was the goal achieved? At the end of 72 hours, do the lesions appear to be healing? Have other problems been identified? Are there revisions to make in the care plan to make it more effective?

When Mrs. Hernandez returned home from work, she continued her assessment and evaluation. Marie's body temperature had continued to rise to 102.2°F and she began to vomit. This must be added to the problem list. What physiological effect could this have on the body? If long lasting, it could affect her comfort, nutrition, and fluid status. The appropriate nursing diagnoses for these risk problems are as follows: *Risk for Altered Nutrition: Less than Body Requirements* and *Risk for Fluid Volume Deficit*. The term *risk* is used because Marie could potentially develop the problematic responses (altered nutrition and fluid deficit) to her illness, although they have not yet occurred.

STUDENT PRACTICE: PROBLEM SOLVING USING THE NURSING PROCESS
Instructions

Read the scenario below and provide answers to the following:

a. List all problem(s).
b. From the problem list, identify one priority nursing diagnosis.
c. Locate and write the definition of the nursing diagnosis.
d. What are *related to* and *as evidenced by* criteria?

1. Terrence Bennet, 8 years old, was brought into the clinic by his grandmother. He presented with multiple lesions on his face and extremities that appeared to be erythematous, ulcerated and moist, with honey-colored crusts. Terrence reported that the lesions itched.

   a. _____
   _____

   b. _____
   _____

   c. _____
   _____

   d. _____
   _____

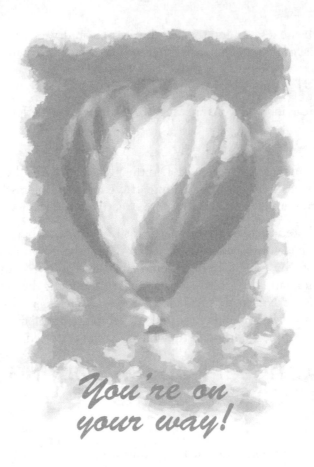

*You're on
your way!*

2. Jay Mullins, 30 years old, was seen in the emergency clinic, after sustaining an injury while playing football. He states he heard a "pop" when he was tackled and is now unable to support weight on his right ankle. He is experiencing pain rated as "8" on a scale of zero to ten. His ankle has severe ecchymosis (bruising) and a large amount of tissue swelling around the fibula.

a. _____

_____

b. _____

_____

c. _____

_____

d. _____

_____

3. Martha Jacob, an 84-year-old female, was seen in her primary care practitioner's office for a check-up two weeks after falling and sustaining a hip injury. She was treated at the time of her injury and released with no broken bones. She was to rest and take one Vicodin every 4 to 6 hours as needed for pain. Although Ms. Jacob reports the pain is somewhat better, her daughter expresses concern that her mother is not eating or drinking fluids well and her stools are hard and infrequent.

   a. _____

   _____

   b. _____

   _____

   c. _____

   _____

   d. _____

   _____

4. Charlotte Maxwell, 66 years old, is waiting to see her primary care physician. She is experiencing the following symptoms: discomfort when she urinates (dysuria), a sense of urgency, she is urinating more frequently, however, voiding only small amounts of urine. Her symptoms have lasted for more than one week and are worsening.

   a. _____

   _____

   b. _____

   _____

   c. _____

   _____

   d. _____

   _____

Assessment

"Assessment, the ability to gather appropriate and pertinent information is considered one of the most important skills that a nurse can develop and possess in caring for the individual patient."

Margarita Valdes, RN, MS (Director, UNITEK College, Vocational Nursing Program, Fremont, California)

STANDARD 1: *ASSESSMENT*

The registered nurse collects comprehensive data pertinent to the patient's health or the situation.

Measurement Criteria

The registered nurse:

- Collects data in a systematic and ongoing process.
- Involves the patient, family, other health care providers, and environment, as appropriate, in holistic data collection.
- Prioritizes data collection activities based on the patient's immediate condition, or anticipated needs of the patient or situation.
- Uses appropriate evidence-based assessment techniques and instruments in collecting pertinent data.
- Uses analytical models and problem-solving tools.
- Synthesizes available data, information, and knowledge relevant to the situation to identify patterns and variances.
- Documents relevant data in a retrievable format.

(From American Nurses Association [2004]. *Nursing: Scope and standards of practice.* Washington, DC: Author.)

OBJECTIVES

Upon completion of this chapter, the student should be able to:

- Identify and describe the components of assessment.
- Differentiate between objective and subjective data.
- Describe the concept of data collection and discuss methods and sources involved in data collection.
- Discuss the importance of establishing a baseline database for comparison of future data.
- Discuss the unique characteristics of the assessment step.
- Identify modes of communication.
- Describe the purpose of therapeutic communication.
- Describe interview preparation and conducting the interview.
- Discuss the three phases of an interview.

KEY TERMS

analyze	inspection	percussion
assessment	interpret	social communication
auscultation	interview	subjective data
baseline data	introduction phase	therapeutic communication
closed question	objective data	validation
closure	observation	verification
data clustering	open-ended question	working phase
holistic	palpation	

ASSESSMENT: STEP 1 OF THE NURSING PROCESS

Assessment is the first step in the nursing process. It involves the act of gathering data about the health status of a client (individual, resident, group of individuals). The information is collected using a systematic approach, then organized, interpreted, verified, and validated to ensure its accuracy.

Finally, data are documented. The care plan is developed from assessment activities, such as the client interview and physical assessment.

Initial data collected become the foundation of the client database and are termed **baseline data.** Thorough and accurate data collection is an important element in planning effective client care. The professional nurse uses deliberate thought processes, judgment, and problem-solving skills as data are compiled.

Data accumulated after the initial assessment are frequently compared to baseline data to determine the client's progress or improvement or to discover trends reflecting deterioration of the client's health status.

Example: Mr. Washington, a 62-year-old African American male, is recovering from hip surgery performed two days ago. According to the previous staff nurse's brief report, he has remained stable throughout the shift. Shortly after report, Mr. Washington becomes anxious and experiences a sudden onset of dyspnea for no apparent reason. Assessment reveals tachycardia, tachypnea, and crackles in bilateral lung bases. Immediately, the nurse reviews baseline and recent vital signs, along with assessment data documented during the past 24-hour nursing record. This change in Mr. Washington's condition is reported without delay to his physician. Further assessment, evaluation, and medical treatment will focus on stabilizing Mr. Washington, transferring him to the intensive care unit, and confirming the complication of pulmonary embolism.

> **Nursing Tip**
>
> *The care plan is developed, based on data gathered from the assessment.*

Characteristics of Assessment

Assessment is the initial step; however, it is systematic, ongoing, and continuous. Assessment is the process of collecting data (information) to identify actual or potential health problems and strengths of the client. The data provides a sense of the client's overall health status. Data collection may include physical, psychological, social, cultural, spiritual, and cognitive areas, as well as developmental level, economic status, functional abilities, and lifestyle, depending on the tool used during data collection.

Data are gathered during an interview, physical examination, and review of diagnostic studies. Information is analyzed and validated, and facts are clustered into groups of information to identify patterns of health or illness. Assessment data are accessible to other health care team members through communication and documentation.

> **Nursing Tip**
>
> *Assessment = data collection, verification, organization, interpretation, and documentation.*

DATA COLLECTION

Data collection begins when the client enters the health care system. The nurse may begin collection prior to initial contact with the client through review of medical records and history. Data collection continues as long as there is a need for health care.

TABLE 2:1 Subjective and Objective Data

Subjective	Objective
• What the person states, e.g., "I'm sad." • These are feelings and perceptions. • "I feel sick to my stomach." • "I wish I were home." • "I have a burning pain in my side." • "I feel like nobody likes me." • "My heart feels like it's racing."	• Things that are observable and measurable by the examiner • Blood pressure of 110/70 • Rash on right arm • Ambulates with a cane • Ate 100% of breakfast • 425 mL clear urine

Types of Data

Data may be separated into two categories, subjective and objective data. **Subjective data,** also known as **symptoms,** are statements, feelings, perceptions, or concerns communicated by a client. For example, "I'm tired" or "I'm having pain" or "I feel so afraid." **Objective data,** also referred to as **signs,** can be observed, measured, or felt by someone other than the person experiencing them. Table 2:1 compares subjective and objective data.

The author recommends that, as novice nurses, students separate collected data into subjective and objective data. Each category will compliment and clarify the other.

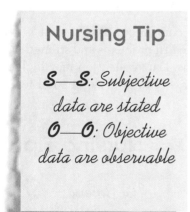

Nursing Tip

S—S: Subjective data are stated

O—O: Objective data are observable

Example:
• Subjective data (what the subject states): "I feel like my heart is racing."
• Objective data: Pulse 150 beats per minute, regular, strong

Objective data usually supports the subjective data. What the nurse observes and measures confirms what the client is feeling and experiencing. However, there may be times when objective data will conflict or seem different from what the client is stating.

Example:
• Subjective data: Client states, "I have no pain."
• Objective data: Color pale, respiratory rate increased from 18 to 26 breaths per minute, clutches abdominal area

In cases where data appear to conflict, the nurse should investigate the situation and gather all pertinent data to understand the problem.

Sources of Data

Gathering data should involve every possible source. However, the client should be the primary source of information, when possible. Family or significant others may provide useful or additional information about the client. Data may be obtained from nursing records, medical records, and verbal or

TABLE 2:2 Subjective and Objective Data Versus Opinions and Conclusions

Subjective Data	Opinion or Conclusion
• "Don't let anyone else in my room."	• Client is angry or hostile.
• "I don't want to have that test."	• Client is anxious.
• "Get this tube out of my nose. It's killing me."	• Client is experiencing pain.
• "How do I get back to my room?"	• Client is disoriented.
• "Why hasn't the doctor seen me today?"	• Client is worried.
Objective Data	**Opinion or Conclusion**
• Dressed and shaved this morning	• Able to attend to ADLs (activities of daily living)
• Unsteady on feet when ambulating	• Client is intoxicated.
• Hands tremble	• Client is afraid or anxious.
• Heart rate 106 beats per minute	• Client is afraid or exercising.
• Client is lying in dark room during the day.	• Client is depressed or sad.
• Voided 300 mL amber urine	• Urine output is adequate.
• Able to change dressing to wound	• Client understands sterile technique.
• Requests pain medication every two hours	• Client is addicted.

written consultations. Other members of the health care team working with the client may provide valuable information. Additional sources include diagnostic results (past and present) and relevant literature, for example, accepted standards (which indicate normal functioning, such as the accepted range of a normal pulse rate).

Data Collection Tools

The assessment database should include all aspects of the client's health status. Assessment tools are designed to help nurses remember what data to collect and to organize the information obtained. Health care facilities develop preprinted documents, which serve as a guide for collecting and recording necessary information. Appendix B contains examples of data collection tools. Most health care facilities use assessment tools based on nursing models considered **holistic**. This term means all aspects of the client's physical, emotional, social, spiritual, and economic well-being are considered (see Figure 2:1). Otherwise, important information relating to how the client lives his or her daily life may be omitted or missed.

Some tools are organized based on problems commonly encountered on a particular nursing unit. For example, pediatric and geriatric data collection tools have additional questions pertaining to these age groups. Any format is acceptable, as long as it is thorough and comprehensive and considers the

Nursing Tip

Just state the facts. Do not state opinions and do not jump to conclusions. See Table 2:2.

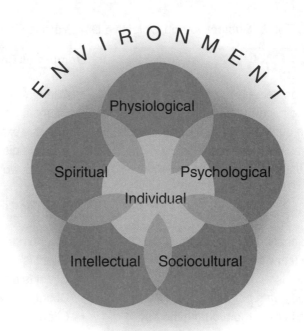

FIGURE 2:1 Holistic perspective of the individual.

client's developmental age. Table 2:3 describes information found on various data collection tools in the client's medical record.

Methods of Data Collection

The nurse collects data through the following methods: observation, interview, and physical assessment.

Observation

The nurse uses observation (the skill of watching thoughtfully and deliberately) to detect the client's overall appearance and behavior. Observations should include physical and emotional responses, moods of the client, and interaction with family or the nurse, as well as social or cultural characteristics, some of which may help or hinder data collection (Figure 2:2). These observations and others are made during initial and subsequent interactions with the client. Table 2:4 provides a checklist to aid in observation techniques.

The ability to communicate is central to the practice of nursing. It is a fundamental element in establishing a restorative nurse-client relationship. Communication includes the ability to appropriately understand, transmit, and receive thoughts, feelings, and facts. In addition, nurses must be aware of cultural differences and variances related to communication. When cultural variances exist, inaccurate interpretation of communication may occur. Table 2:5 describes ways of overcoming possible cultural communication barriers.

TABLE 2:3 Medical Record Documents

Document	Information
Face sheet	Biographical data: name, date of birth, address, phone number, Social Security number, marital status, employment, race, gender, religion, closest relative, insurance coverage, allergies, attending physician, admitting medical diagnosis, assigned diagnosis-related group, statement of whether the client has an advance directive.
Consent form	Admit: gives the institution and physician the right to treat. Surgery: explains the reason for the operation in lay terms, the risks for complications, and the client's level of understanding. Blood transfusion: permission to administer blood or blood products.
Medical history and physical examination	Results of the client's initial history and physical assessment as performed by the health care provider.
Prescriber order sheet	Medical orders to admit and the treatment plan.
Progress notes	Evaluation of the client's response to treatment; may contain the progress recording of interdisciplinary practitioners (e.g., dietary or social services).
Consultation sheet	Initiated by the physician to request the evaluation or services of other practitioners.
Diagnostic sheet	Contains the results from laboratory and diagnostic tests (e.g., radiograph, hematology).
Nursing admit assessment	Recording of data obtained from the interview and physical assessment conducted by the RN.
Nursing plan of care	Contains the treatment plan (e.g., nursing diagnosis or a problem list, initiation of standards of care or protocols).
Graphic sheet	Data recording regarding vital signs and weight.
Flow sheet	Contains all routine interventions that can be noted with a check mark or other simple code; allows for a quick comparison of measurement.

(continues)

TABLE 2:3 Medical Record Documents (*continued*)

Document	Information
Nurse's progress notes	Additional data that do not duplicate information on the flow sheet (e.g., client's achievement of expected outcome or revision of the plan of care).
Medication administration record	Contains all medication information for routine and prn (as needed) drugs: date, time, dose, route, site (for injections).
Patient education record	Recording of the nurses' teaching of the client, family, or other caregiver and the learner's response.
Health care team record	Treatment and progress record for nonmedical and nonnursing practitioners, when the physician's progress notes are not used by other practitioners (e.g., respiratory, physical therapy, dietary).
Clinical pathway	A multidisciplinary form for each day of anticipated hospitalization that identifies the interventions and achievement of client outcomes; the practitioner's initial implementation and variances from the norm are explained in the progress notes.
Discharge plan and summary	A multidisciplinary form used before discharge from a health care facility containing a brief summary of care rendered and discharge instructions (e.g., food-drug interactions, referrals, or follow-up appointments).
Advance directive or living will	Federal law requires that health care providers discuss with clients the use of advance directives, commonly known as the living will or durable power of attorney. Most states recognize the living will as a legal document. If the client has advance directives, they are reviewed at the time of admission and placed in the medical record.

Adapted from Delaune, Sue C., & Ladner, Patricia K. (2002). *Fundamentals of nursing: Standards and practice* (2nd ed.) New York: Thomson Delmar Learning.

Interview

An **interview** is a communication exchange between the client and nurse. This exchange has a specific purpose, which is to collect information about the client. Discoveries relating to the client's present and past health status allow the nurse to make determinations and decisions about health needs. Nurses use

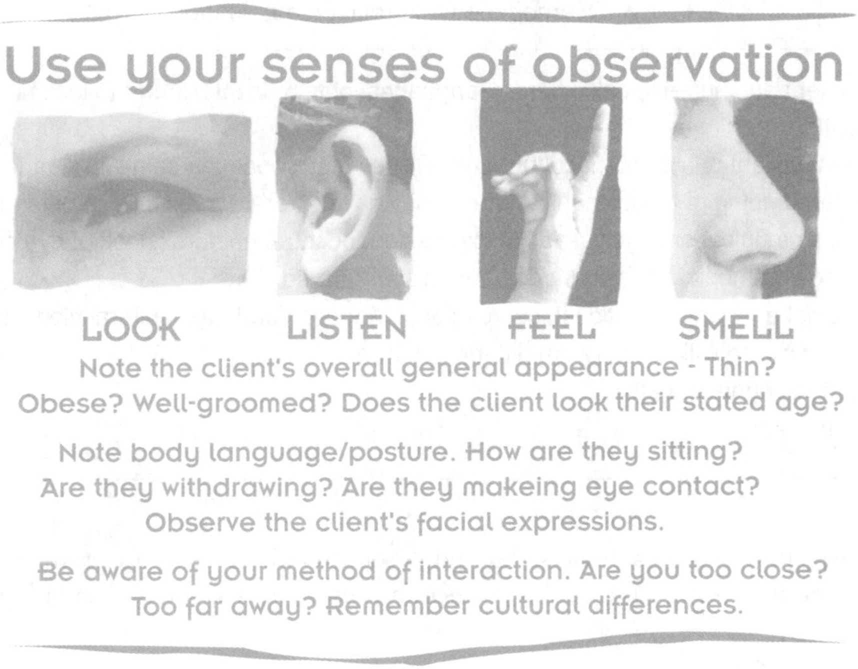

Use your senses of observation

LOOK   LISTEN   FEEL   SMELL

Note the client's overall general appearance - Thin?
Obese? Well-groomed? Does the client look their stated age?

Note body language/posture. How are they sitting?
Are they withdrawing? Are they makeing eye contact?
Observe the client's facial expressions.

Be aware of your method of interaction. Are you too close?
Too far away? Remember cultural differences.

FIGURE 2:2

knowledge of communication to discerningly obtain facts and information. This information is gathered through conversation and observations during the structured interview. Developing interviewing skills takes time and practice.

There are different types of communication: therapeutic and social. For the purpose of data collection, the nurse uses **therapeutic communication.** This interaction results in conversations with a client

TABLE 2:4 Aids to Observation

- Use your senses _____
- Note the client's general appearance _____
  _____
- Note body language _____
  _____
- Be aware of own interaction patterns _____
  Remember cultural differences relating to behavior

TABLE 2:5 Overcoming Cultural Communication Barriers

- When the client and nurse speak different languages, obtain an interpreter to facilitate communication.
- Even though a client of a different culture and a nurse may speak the same language, verify the client's understanding of the exchange. Words may have different meanings to different people.
- Nonverbal communication, such as facial expression, posture, gestures, lack of eye contact, and use of silence are communication variances often misinterpreted.
- Consider social and family relationships, religion, language, food, and cultural view of health or illness when working with clients from differing cultures.
- Maintain a nonjudgmental attitude.
- Recognize biases.

which are neither idle nor meaningless, but purposeful, goal-directed, focused on the client, and planned. **Social communication** is casual conversation, spontaneous, and with no planned agenda.

Nursing Tip

People differ in many ways:
- Age
- Gender
- Educational level
- Language
- Occupation
- Residence (rural, urban, suburban)
- Socioeconomic status
- Religion
- Functional abilities
- Cognitive abilities
- Racial composition
- Nationality
- Family structure and ties

Interview Preparation

Preparation and planning are key to effective interviewing. Suggestions for preparation include reviewing medical records, reviewing current admission documentation of past or present client care, and researching present and past medical diagnoses. In addition, forethought should be given to strategies for overcoming potential communication barriers which might impede successful data collection during the interview process. Table 2:6 identifies common barriers to therapeutic interaction.

TABLE 2:6 Barriers to Therapeutic Interaction

Barrier	Example
• Language differences	• Difficulty navigating through health care system. • Prevents evaluation of client's response to nursing interventions.
• Sociocultural differences	• Use of language may differ from nurse. Interpretation of words may be different.
• Gender	• Communication can vary between men and women.
• Health status	• The disoriented or confused client is unable to reliably communicate. • Alterations in sensory or perceptual function, such as impairment or loss of vision, hearing, or sense of touch, affect the ability to send or receive communication messages. • Moderate to severe pain or discomfort and other health-related difficulties, such as dyspnea, may impair communication.
• Developmental level	• May require a different approach, different language, or different terminology in order for a client (for example, a child) to understand.
• Knowledge differences	• Client and family may have varying levels of education. Listen to conversations and vocabulary chosen. Consider the client's mental capabilities.
• Emotional distance	• Therapeutic communication involves establishing a caring, empathetic relationship with the client. Emotional distance refers to a barrier existing between the client and nurse which prevents effective therapeutic communication. Examples include a client in respiratory isolation or a comatose or confused client.
• Emotions	• Fear, anxiety, and depression are examples of emotions that prevent therapeutic communication.
• Daydreaming	• Allowing one's mind to wander instead of being an active listener may lead to missing the point of the message. Nurses must be attentive, alert, and focused on the conversation.

Conducting the Interview

The interview most often occurs at the beginning of the nurse-client relationship. The nurse may institute various techniques in an effort to build rapport with the client (Figure 2:3). Rapport promotes positive interactions between the health care team and client.

Techniques that advocate productive, therapeutic communication include: active listening, conveying acceptance, being attentive, sitting at eye level with the client, if possible, and establishing eye-to-eye contact.

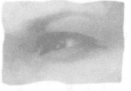

Tips to help you establish rapport with the client

MAINTAIN EYE CONTACT

1. Interview in a private setting - environment should be quiet, private. Turn down the TV. Close the room door.

2. When addressing the client, use appropriate title. Introduce yourself.

3. State the purpose of the exchange/interview. Explain why you will be asking questions.

4. Maintain eye contact - do not stare, but be attentive.

5. Do not rush through the data collection tool. Use a caring, interested manner, clarifying and investigating, when appropriate.

FIGURE 2:3

Controlling the environment, making it more conducive for the interview, is an important part of preparation. This includes providing privacy, allowing adequate time for answering questions, maintaining a comfortable room temperature, reducing environmental noise levels, and eliminating or decreasing distractions, if possible.

There are three phases to an interview: introduction, working, and closure. During the **introduction phase** of the interview, goals for the interaction are stated. Both the purpose and use of collected data should be discussed. For example, the nurse might begin by stating, "I need to ask you a few questions about your health, so I can better plan for your care." Inform the client how long the interview will last.

The **working phase** of the interview focuses on the details of data collection. The assessment interview may consist of collecting comprehensive data, for example, a detailed past medical history, as well as a thorough physical examination. An assessment interview may also be focused on a specific area, such as data collection regarding pain description. Specific data collection tool formats are used during the assessment interview and will aid in data organization. The tool will depend on the type of information to be collected and the model accepted and used by the facility.

Data collection is facilitated by various communication techniques. During the interview, nurses ask questions to elicit a particular response. How questions are asked will determine client responses (Figure 2:4). **Open-ended questions** are stated in a manner that encourages the client to elaborate about a particular concern or problem. For example, "What types of food do you usually eat during a

Interviewing Techniques

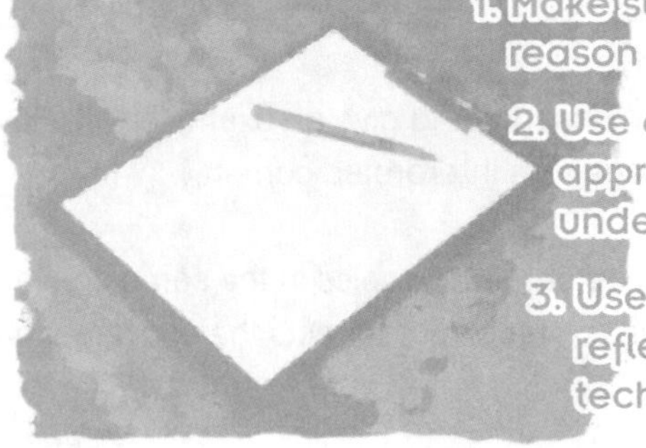

1. Make sure your questions are relevant to the reason the client is seeking health care.

2. Use correct terminology - remember age appropriate terms and use terms the client can understand. Do not talk down to the client.

3. Use open-ended questions and comments, reflection, summarize, restate...communication techniques.

4. Use an organized, systematic assessment tool.

FIGURE 2:4

twenty-four-hour period?" or "What led to your coming here today?" Each of these questions encourages the client to respond with information. Closed questions can be answered with brief yes-or-no answers. This type of questioning may be appropriate in certain situations, for example, in an emergency: "Did she respond to you when you entered her room?" or "How many pounds has she lost over the last month?" Additional techniques that promote communication during an interview or therapeutic nurse-client communication can be found in Table 2:7 and Figure 2:5.

Bringing Closure to the Interview

The nurse should indicate in some manner that the interview session is coming to an end. For example, the nurse could state that most of the information has been collected and only a few more facts are necessary. During closure, the nurse allows the client to present additional relevant information and then summarizes overall information that has been covered or accomplished. The nurse determines if additional sessions will be necessary for further exploration and, if so, plans are made with the client.

Physical Examination

The purpose of a physical examination is to collect data regarding the client's present health status and to establish a baseline physical assessment. Direct observations can be made which may indicate deviations from normal. Validation and clarification of any subjective complaints may be obtained.

TABLE 2:7 Therapeutic Communication Techniques

Paraphrasing	Restate what was said by the sender in the receiver's own words to make sure the statement was understood accurately.
Clarifying	Asking the sender to restate an unclear message or to give an example will allow confirmation of whether or not the message was interpreted correctly.
Focusing	When the sender introduces more than one unrelated topics in the same conversation or when the discussion becomes unclear, the receiver redirects the conversation back to a specific topic.
Summarizing	Reviewing a conversation and focusing on key issues provides a synopsis of the main ideas from the discussion.
Responses and actions to avoid	• Inattentive listening, such as breaking eye contact, glancing around the room, or fidgeting, conveys the message that what the sender has to say is not important. • Using unfamiliar medical terminology may be confusing to the patient and family. • Asking unrelated personal questions simply to satisfy your curiosity is inappropriate. • Providing false reassurance may discourage expression of feelings. • Inappropriate socializing borders on unprofessional behavior and blocks therapeutic communication. • Passive responses sidestep subject matter or conflict. • Aggressive responses trigger conflict.

Promoting a Successful Interview

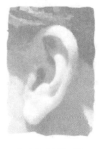

1. Listen actively! Convey acceptance - make eye contact, nod your head to show interest. Be attentive - concentrate on the client's words.

2. Allow client/family member to finish sentences/thoughts - don't interrupt.

3. Be patient - allow time for client to answer or respond.

LISTEN!

4. When appropriate, summarize and restate.

FIGURE 2:5

Nursing Tip

- *Always promote communication while assessing.*
- *Ask questions and then allow time for response.*
- *Do not rely on memory. Write it down.*
- *Choose a method for organizing your assessment, e.g., head to toe, body systems.*

During a physical examination, the nurse uses various techniques to collect data. Initial physical data collected, known as baseline data, are documented and used for comparison and evaluation of the client's status at a given point in time.

Physical Examination Techniques

Physical assessment techniques include *inspection, auscultation, palpation,* and *percussion.* A brief description of each technique follows.

Inspection is a systematic process of observation that includes vision. Through sight, the nurse observes skin color and condition, notes drainage, the effort to breathe, and respiratory pattern. Inspection includes noting one's body posture, gait, ability to use extremities, and facial expressions or observing the client's ability to carry out activities of daily living (ADLs).

- Use a penlight or natural or artificial lighting to enhance inspection.
- Maintain privacy during inspection and throughout all phases of the physical examination.
- Explain the inspection technique to the client prior to beginning to reduce anxiety.

Auscultation is the technique of listening for sounds within the body, usually with a stethoscope. Areas most often auscultated include lungs, heart, abdomen, and blood vessels.

Palpation is an assessment technique involving use of touch or pressing on the external surface of the body with the fingers. Palpation is used to assess texture, temperature, moisture of the skin, organ location and size, vibrations and pulsations, swelling, masses, and tenderness. Examples of uses of palpation include:

- Touch: may be used to detect a mass, conditions of the skin, e.g., moisture, dryness, skin temperature
- Pressure: may be employed to feel the quality and rate of an arterial pulsation, to determine capillary refill, assess skin turgor, or to evaluate for edema
- Deep palpation: may be used for assessment of deep, internal organ anomalies or to determine if the client is experiencing an abnormal response to pain

Percussion is the technique involving direct or indirect tapping of a specific body surface to glean information about internal organs beneath the body surface. The health care provider may use fingertips, fist, or percussion hammer to elicit various tones indicating presence or absence of fluid or air, masses, consolidation, tenderness, and normal or abnormal reflexes.

Nursing Tip

Roles of the Nurse:
- Caregiver
- Counselor
- Teacher
- Client advocate
- Change agent
- Team member
- Resource person

DATA VERIFICATION AND VALIDATION

After all data are gathered, information is **verified** (confirmed or proved) and **validated** (determined to be fact) to ensure accuracy. Data are reviewed for omissions, inconsistencies, or possible inaccuracies. For example, a confused client is admitted to the medical surgical unit, stating that he has no family. However, you were told that the person who brought him in was his wife. In another example, a client may state that he ambulates without difficulty and without the use of assistive devices. The client's wife states he uses a cane. The nurse observes the client ambulating with an unsteady gait. In each case, the nurse would need to consider possible reasons for the discrepancy and collect more information before forming conclusions and planning care.

Nursing Tip

Identify problems by asking the following questions:
1. Has the client experienced any change in his or her usual functional pattern?
2. Has the client demonstrated any indication of abnormal functioning of a body system?
3. Has the client demonstrated deviation from normal range when compared to standards?

INTERPRETATION AND ORGANIZATION OF DATA

Data which have been collected, verified, and validated for accuracy are now ready to be **analyzed** (processing information to reach a conclusion) and **interpreted** (determining the meaning and significance). For this process, the nurse assigns meaning to collected data and groups data into clusters. Data are compared against standards such as normal health patterns, normal vital signs, lab values, basic food groups, or normal growth and development. Interpreting and analyzing data help identify missing information or inconsistencies. Once these are identified, it would be necessary to gather more data.

Data clustering is the process of organizing subjective and objective data into groups of related cues. This process is used to determine the relatedness of facts, to find patterns, and to determine if further data are needed. Ultimately, data clustering assists in identifying areas of health care deviations requiring treatment or support.

Example:
1. "Reports sudden onset of abdominal pain rated six on a scale of zero to ten, observed facial mask of pain, guarding abdominal area," are clustered data indicating acute pain as a nursing diagnosis.
2. "Reports difficulty carrying out ADLs, observed difficulty dressing self and brushing hair," are clustered data indicating problems with self-care abilities.
3. "Uses a walker, has difficulty ambulating, stumbles and looses balance when attempts to ambulate to bathroom," are clustered data indicating problems with mobility.

DOCUMENTING ASSESSMENT DATA

Documentation of data collected during the assessment is essential. Documentation is the process of preparing a record that reflects the assessment data and describes the client's present health status. When documenting this information, the nurse communicates with others involved in the client's care. This is necessary to provide quality care.

Various formats are utilized for documentation, depending on the agency. Data may be documented using narrative notations, checklists, a combination of the two, or specialty formats. Chapter 5 discusses and describes different types of documentation. Appendix B includes examples of assessment data collection tools and documentation forms.

KEY CONCEPTS

- Assessment is the first step in the nursing process. Information is gathered through an interview, physical examination, and review of diagnostic tests. These data reveal a sense of the overall health status of the client.
- Assessment is ongoing throughout the nursing process sequence.
- During assessment, data are collected, organized, interpreted, verified, validated, and then documented.
- The care plan is developed from and based on data collected during initial and ongoing assessment.
- Two types of data are collected: subjective and objective. Generally, each category will complement and clarify the other.
- The client should be the primary source of information. When this is not possible, family or significant others may provide useful or additional information about the client.

- Data sources include the client, nursing records, medical records, verbal and written consultations, diagnostic results, and relevant literature.
- Methods of data collection include observation, interview, and physical examination.
- Collected data should be verified and validated to ensure accuracy. Data should be reviewed for omissions and incongruities. If these are discovered, possible reasons for the discrepancy or inaccuracy should be identified and corrected.
- Clustering helps to organize data and determine the *relatedness* of subjective and objective information. Clustering also aids in finding patterns. This technique provides confirmation that an identified problem exists and should be included in the care plan.

STUDENT PRACTICE: DEVELOPING COMMUNICATION AND DATA COLLECTION
Instructions

Provide responses to the following:

1. Define baseline database and explain its importance. _____
   _____
   _____

2. Define subjective and objective data. Provide an example of each. _____
   _____
   _____

3. List characteristics of therapeutic communication. _____
   _____
   _____

4. Describe communication techniques that promote therapeutic communication. _____
   _____
   _____

5. Explain the role of the interview, observation, and physical assessment in data collection. ____
   _____
   _____
   _____

6. List key elements of a successful interview. _____
   _____
   _____

STUDENT PRACTICE: DEVELOPING OPEN-ENDED QUESTIONS

Instructions

Transform the following "closed" questions to open-ended questions or comments to promote therapeutic communication.

1. "Are you feeling better?"

_____

_____

2. "Did you like the dinner?"

_____

_____

3. "Are you in pain?"

_____

_____

4. "Do you understand what the doctor told you about the surgery?"

_____

_____

5. "Do you understand the doctor's instructions?"

_____

_____

STUDENT PRACTICE: DEVELOPING THERAPEUTIC COMMUNICATION TECHNIQUES

Instructions

Rewrite the following quotes using specified therapeutic communication techniques:

1. The client comments, "Nothing ever goes right for me." Use reflection and write your response.

_____

_____

_____

2. The client is extremely quiet and avoids eye contact. Use observation and write your response.

_____

_____

_____

3. The client states, "They told me I had to have surgery. I'm so afraid. I couldn't sleep last night. I'm waiting for my husband to call me from home. He had to pick up the kids. Right now, I have a headache." Use focusing and write your response. _____

_____

_____

4. The client states, "I felt full even before I started eating." Use clarifying and write your response.

_____

_____

_____

STUDENT PRACTICE: IDENTIFYING OBJECTIVE AND SUBJECTIVE DATA

Instructions

Underline _abnormal_ data discovered in the situations below. List subjective and objective data.

Scenario: Cherisha Martin, a 56-year-old African American female, was seen at the clinic with multiple urinary system complaints. She reports that her urine is cloudy, amber colored, and has a pungent odor. She has an urge to urinate more frequently, however she voids small amounts. Two days ago, she saw blood in her urine. Her vital signs are: blood pressure 142/92, pulse rate 78 per minute and regular, respirations 20 breaths per minute, and temperature 100.4°F.

1. List abnormal subjective data from the case scenario above.

_____

_____

_____

2. List abnormal objective data from the case scenario above.

_____

_____

_____

Scenario: Richardo Gutierrez, a 34-year-old Hispanic male, was involved in a roll-over motor vehicle accident one day ago. In the accident, he sustained a crushing injury to his right hand. He has multiple superficial cuts from broken glass on his arms and face. This morning he describes his hand pain as throbbing and deep. He rates his pain as "six" on a zero to ten scale. The dressing on his hand is intact with a small amount of dry, reddish-brown drainage observed in the palmar region. His fingertips are edematous, warm, with a brisk capillary refill. His radial pulse is palpable and within normal limits.

1. List abnormal subjective data from the case scenario above.

   _____

   _____

   _____

2. List abnormal objective data from the case scenario above.

   _____

   _____

   _____

Diagnosis

"A clinical judgment about individual, family, or community responses to actual and potential health problems/life processes, nursing diagnoses provide the basis for selection of nursing interventions to achieve outcomes for which the nurse is accountable."

NANDA

STANDARD 2: *DIAGNOSIS*

The registered nurse analyzes assessment data to determine diagnoses or issues.

Measurement Criteria

The registered nurse:

- Derives diagnoses or issues based on assessment data.
- Validates diagnoses or issues with the patient, family, and other health care providers when possible and appropriate.
- Documents diagnoses or issues in a manner that facilitates the determination of the expected outcomes and plan.

(From American Nurses Association. [2004]. *Nursing: Scope and standards of practice.* Washington, DC: Author.)

OBJECTIVES

Upon completion of this chapter, the student should be able to:

- Identify characteristics of nursing diagnoses.
- Identify and discuss differences between medical and nursing diagnoses.

- Describe the different types of nursing diagnoses.
- List components of actual and risk nursing diagnoses.
- Describe the process of developing a nursing diagnosis.

KEY TERMS

actual nursing diagnosis
defining characteristics
diagnosis
etiology

medical diagnosis
nursing diagnosis
problem
problem statement

risk nursing diagnosis
wellness diagnosis

DIAGNOSIS: STEP 2 OF THE NURSING PROCESS

Diagnosis is the second phase of the nursing process. It involves the classification of disease, condition, or human response based upon scientific evaluation of signs, symptoms, history, and diagnostic studies. Diagnosis is also referred to as analysis, problem identification, or nursing diagnosis. These corresponding terms are used interchangeably.

During the assessment phase, nurses use critical-thinking skills and judgment to analyze, organize, and interpret assessment data. Problems, potential problems, and strengths of the client are identified. In the diagnosis phase, problems, potential problems, and strengths are labeled with an appropriate nursing diagnosis. Once labeled, the nursing diagnosis communicates specific health care needs about the client to other members of the health care team involved in care.

Nursing Tip

All activities preceding this phase are directed toward formulating the nursing diagnosis, that is, problem identification. All care planning activities following this phase are based on the nursing diagnosis, the identified problem(s).

Differentiating Between Medical and Nursing Diagnoses

A medical diagnosis is made by the physician or advance health care practitioner and refers to a disease, condition, or pathological state only a practitioner can treat. Examples of medical diagnoses are diabetes mellitus, congestive heart failure, hepatitis, cancer, and pneumonia. The medical diagnosis usually does not change. Nurses are required to follow the physician's order(s) and carry out prescribed treatments and therapies.

The term *nursing diagnosis* is used in three different contexts. First, it refers to the distinct second step in the nursing process, diagnosis. Next, nursing diagnosis applies to the label. Nurses assign meaning to collected assessment data. Actual problems and problems the client is at risk for developing are identified and appropriately labeled with a NANDA-approved nursing diagnosis. For example, a client is admitted into the hospital and medically treated for a heart attack (acute myocardial infarction). The physician prescribes treatment, such as diagnostic tests, therapies, and various medications. The nurse carries out the physician orders and monitors the client. During the assessment, the nurse may identify that the client is experiencing anxiety over the medical diagnosis, fear and anxiety over an uncertain future, and difficulty sleeping. It is those problems which are labeled with nursing diagnoses: respectively, *Anxiety, Fear,* and *Sleep Pattern Disturbed.* Nurses will intervene individually or collectively with the physician to resolve each response. Nurses understand the holistic needs of the client and use scientific knowledge, insight, and critical thought as physician-prescribed treatment and nursing interventions are carried out. Finally, a nursing diagnosis refers to one of many diagnoses in the classification system established and approved by NANDA. A complete list of nursing diagnoses, NANDA taxonomy, can be found in Appendix A.

Characteristics of Nursing Diagnoses

Actual nursing diagnoses describe the client's response to a physical, sociocultural, psychological, and/or spiritual illness, disease, or condition. Actual signs and symptoms are present. For example, the physician diagnoses a client with a medical illness, pneumonia, and writes orders for hospital admission and treatment. During the initial interview and assessment, subjective and objective data are collected indicating the client is restless, hypoxic (reduced oxygen in inspired air), and too weak to cough productively. The nurse correctly identifies and labels one nursing diagnosis as *Impaired Gas Exchange.* Interventions will be planned and instituted by the nurse to improve the client's gas exchange at the cellular level, aiding in problem improvement or resolution.

Nursing diagnoses may communicate possible developing problems resulting from a client's physical, sociocultural, psychological, and/or spiritual illness, disease, or condition, termed risk nursing diagnoses. For example, an elderly client experiencing vertigo and difficulty walking refuses to call for assistance with ambulation. The appropriate potential problem would be identified and labeled as *Risk for Injury.*

Nursing diagnoses may change as the client's condition improves or the problem resolves or becomes worse. Refer back to the example of the client diagnosed with *Impaired Gas Exchange.* Nurses carry out physician-prescribed treatment for pneumonia, e.g., administer antibiotics, provide hydration, etc., and the client's physical condition improves. One would expect gas exchange within the lungs to improve. In this case, the problem of *Impaired Gas Exchange* would probably be resolved.

Nursing diagnoses may compliment physician-prescribed treatment, but are separate and distinct. For example, if the hospitalized client had undergone a surgical procedure, one would expect to find

TABLE 3:1 Determining Appropriate Interventions Using Critical Thought

Mrs. Johnson, sixty-six years of age, is admitted after falling and fracturing her pelvis. Data are gathered through an interview and physical assessment. The client requests medication for pain. The pain she is experiencing is a physiological response to her injury. Using a NANDA nursing diagnosis, the response is labeled as *Acute Pain.*

Mrs. Johnson's physician has written analgesic orders, as follows:
- Demerol 50 mg, intramuscular, every four hours, as needed for severe pain
- Vicodin one or two, by mouth, every four hours, as needed for moderate pain
- Tylenol ES two, by mouth every four hours, as needed for mild pain

What decision-making questions should the nurse ask Mrs. Johnson regarding her pain?

Nursing Tip

A client's medical diagnosis remains the same for as long as the disease process is present, whereas nursing diagnoses often change as the client's responses change.

physician-ordered analgesics. Medication is one important method to treat pain. (See Table 3:1, which shows an example of an analgesic order that a physician would write.) There are also many independent nonpharmacological nursing interventions which may be initiated to alleviate the client's pain, and which would complement physician-prescribed treatment. Examples include imagery, distraction, relaxation, and massage.

Actual nursing diagnoses are developed when an *existing response* to an illness, disease, or condition is present at the time of the nursing assessment. The problem actually exists. The client is demonstrating subjective and/or objective data to support the conclusion. Actual nursing diagnoses are based on the presence of associated signs and symptoms.

Example:
Hyperthermia, client's temperature is 104.6°F
Impaired Gas Exchange, client's oxygen saturation in arterial blood is 92%
Pain, client states pain level is "eight" on scale of zero to ten
Anxiety, client states he is experiencing anxiety
Self-Care Deficit, client is unable to perform ADLs

Risk diagnoses are determined when a possible problem may develop but has not yet occurred. NANDA defines risk diagnosis as "a clinical judgment made when a client is more vulnerable to develop the problem than others in the same or similar situations."

Example:
Any person admitted into the hospital is at risk for acquiring a nosocomial infection. However, a client medically diagnosed with cancer, who is receiving chemotherapy and whose immune system is depressed, will hold a higher risk than others will for developing a hospital-acquired infection. The nurse would appropriately label this potential problem as *Risk for Infection*. Once identified, the health care team can take deliberate action and initiate interventions to prevent the problem from occurring.

Example:
An active 80-year-old female was admitted into the hospital two days ago after falling in her home and sustaining a pelvic fracture. Day one after surgical repair, the client is experiencing a great deal of pain and refuses to move. Immobility, advanced age, and the client's refusal to shift her weight place the client at a greater risk for developing pressure ulcers. The nurse appropriately labels this potential problem as *Risk for Impaired Skin Integrity* and plans interventions to prevent skin breakdown from occurring.

Nursing Tip
- *The same set of nursing diagnoses cannot be expected to occur with a particular disease or condition.*
- *A single nursing diagnosis may occur as a response to any number of diseases.*

Components of Actual Nursing Diagnoses

For *actual* nursing diagnoses, the **problem statement** consists of three components: problem, etiology, and defining characteristics. Each element has a specific purpose.

The **problem** is the identified label of a client's health condition or response to the medical illness or therapy for which nursing may intervene. The problem is also known as the nursing diagnosis.

The **etiology,** written 'as related to' (R/T) includes conditions most likely to be involved in the development of a problem. This factor becomes the focus for nursing interventions. The etiology or cause component of the nursing diagnosis identifies one or more probable causes of the abnormal response. The etiology gives direction to the problem statement. In view of this fact, the nurse is able to individualize care. NANDA uses the term *related factor* to describe the etiology or likely cause of the actual nursing diagnosis.

Defining characteristics, written 'as evidenced by' (AEB), are the clinical signs and symptoms which confirm the problem exists. This component reflects *how* the diagnosis or problematic response is manifested.

Nursing Tip

Remember, for actual nursing diagnoses, there are subjective and/or objective data, evidence that the problem actually exists.

Student Practice Examples

The following scenarios describe patient situations in which clinical signs and symptoms resulting from their illness, condition, or injury are exhibited. The actual nursing diagnosis is provided.

A. Using Appendix A, locate the nursing diagnosis and read the definition.
B. List all appropriate 'related to' and 'as evidenced by' components.

Scenario one: The nurse is caring for a client who was involved in a motor vehicle accident and sustained superficial skin trauma. The client's epidermal layer of skin on the right knee, forearm, and hand is excoriated, reddened, and bleeding as the result of sliding across a cement pavement. (Impaired Skin Integrity)

_____

_____

_____

_____

_____

Scenario two: Carson, a two-year-old male, has had a productive cough for three days. His respiratory rate is increased for his age and he is irritable. Carson is diagnosed with acute bronchitis and placed on antibiotics and home breathing treatments. (*Impaired Gas Exchange*)

_____

_____

_____

_____

Scenario three: The client you are caring for has been medically diagnosed with a right cerebral vascular accident (stroke). He experiences partial paralysis on the left side of his body. He is unable to turn over while in bed without assistance and has demonstrated decreased muscle strength and control in the left extremities. (*Impaired Physical Mobility*)

_____

_____

_____

_____

_____

Nursing Tip

Differentiating among possible causes of an identified problem is essential. Each cause or etiology may require different nursing interventions (see Table 3:2).

Components of Risk Nursing Diagnoses

Risk nursing diagnoses are identified when the client is *at risk* for developing a problem. The problem statement consists of two components, the problem and risk factor. The term *risk factor* is used to describe the etiology of risk nursing diagnoses, because there are no subjective or objective data present. The actual problem *does not exist* at the time of assessment. However, due to clinical circumstances, the client is at risk for developing this specific problem or complication. Table 3:3 compares components of actual and risk nursing diagnoses.

Examples of Risk Nursing Diagnoses

- Cancer patient, *Risk for Infection*
  R/T: inadequate secondary defenses, immunosuppression
- Client with surgical incision, *Risk for Infection*
  R/T: inadequate primary defenses, invasive procedure
- Client who is semiconscious, vomiting, *Risk for Aspiration*
  R/T: reduced level of consciousness, vomiting

TABLE 3:2 Comparison of Same Nursing Diagnoses with Different Etiologies Requiring Different Interventions

Nursing Diagnosis	Client	Etiology	Nursing Interventions
Constipation, Perceived	Jim Beason	Inactivity, insufficient fiber intake	• Encourage daily activity to stimulate bowel elimination • Teach components of high-fiber diet to improve bowel function
	Terry Fielder	Long-term laxative use	• Identify factors that may contribute to constipation, such as medications, reduced fluid intake, dietary habits • Instruct client on adverse effects of long-term laxative use
Ineffective breast-feeding	Christi Lawrence	Inadequate sucking reflex in infant	• Assess infant's ability to latch on and suck effectively • Monitor maternal skill with latching infant onto the nipple
	Cheri Phillips	Inexperience, knowledge deficit	• Determine mother's desire and motivation to breast-feed • Evaluate mother's understanding of infant's feeding cues, such as rooting

TABLE 3:3 Comparison of Components in Actual and Risk Nursing Diagnoses

Actual Nursing Diagnosis	Risk Nursing Diagnosis
Three components: • Nursing diagnosis • Related factor(s) • Defining characteristics	Two components: • Risk nursing diagnosis • Risk factor(s)

Nursing Tip

For risk nursing diagnoses, there are no defining characteristics or AEB, per se. R/T identify characteristics that make the client more vulnerable to developing a specific problem.

- Neonate unable to maintain his body temperature, parent does not keep the child covered, *Risk for Hypothermia*
  R/T: extremes of age, inadequate clothing
- Unsteady gait, refuses to call for assistance, *Risk for Injury*
  R/T: impaired mobility, lack of knowledge regarding safety precautions

Wellness Nursing Diagnoses

NANDA defines wellness diagnosis as "a clinical judgment about an individual, family, or community in transition from a specific level of wellness to a higher level of wellness." Wellness nursing diagnoses require a one-part statement, for example, Readiness for Enhanced Nutrition (client has expressed a desire for improved nutritional status).

KEY CONCEPTS

- Diagnosis is the second step in the nursing process.
- Nursing diagnoses are different than medical diagnoses, in that nursing diagnoses describe the *client's response* to a physical, sociocultural, psychological, or spiritual illness, disease, or condition.
- Nurses have legal and ethical responsibilities to both medical and nursing diagnoses.
- Nursing diagnoses may change as the client's health status changes.
- The two most common nursing diagnoses are *actual* and *risk for* nursing diagnoses.
- An actual nursing diagnosis includes three components: the problem (nursing diagnosis label), etiology (related to), and defining characteristics (as evidenced by).
- A risk nursing diagnosis includes two components: the potential problem (risk nursing diagnosis) and risk factors (related to).
- Wellness nursing diagnoses require a one-part statement. Wellness nursing diagnoses may be included in the care plan for individuals expressing desire for a higher level of wellness.

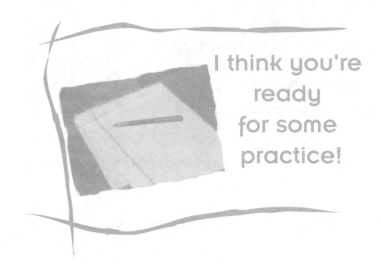

I think you're ready for some practice!

STUDENT PRACTICE: WRITING DIAGNOSIS STATEMENTS
Instructions

Read each case history and follow directions.

A. *Underline* abnormal subjective data and *circle* abnormal objective data.
B. Complete the *three-part* diagnostic statement that clearly describes the nursing diagnosis. In other words, what is the *R/T* and *AEB* information you will include with the nursing diagnosis?

1. Carl James was hospitalized yesterday. Today he demonstrates the following signs and symptoms: blood pressure 138/78, pulse rate 102 per minute and regular, respiratory rate 24 per minute and using accessory muscles, restless, and irritable. Oral temperature is 99.8°F. The pulse oximeter reading is 94%. Mr. James is diaphoretic and complains of a headache. His lung sounds are clear, but diminished. He states he feels "light-headed" when he moves from his bed to the chair. (Nursing diagnosis, *Impaired Gas Exchange*)

   _____

   _____

   _____

   _____

2. Mrs. Silverman has recently completed chemotherapy and radiation for breast cancer. She arrived at the clinic this morning with the following signs and symptoms: no appetite, weight loss of four pounds since her last visit two weeks ago, nausea, however, no vomiting. She states most of the time she feels exhausted. "The inside of my mouth hurts." Assessment reveals oral ulcerations which are

erythematous (reddened). Her vital signs are within normal range. (Nursing diagnosis, *Imbalanced Nutrition: Less Than Body Requirements*)

_____

_____

_____

_____

3. Kam Le returned from South America one week ago. He has experienced nausea, vomiting and diarrhea for four days and exhibits the following additional symptoms: inelastic skin turgor, dry oral mucous membranes, weakness, and an elevated temperature. (Nursing diagnosis, *Fluid Volume Deficient*)

_____

_____

_____

_____

4. Seventy-seven-year-old Hilda Jameson, is being evaluated at the clinic. Her daughter states Mrs. Jamison has not been as active as usual and has experienced frequent episodes of confusion. Examination confirms she is disoriented to time and place and asks that someone find her husband. Her daughter reports that he has been deceased for several years. (Nursing diagnosis, *Disturbed Thought Processes*)

_____

_____

_____

_____

_____

_____

STUDENT PRACTICE: IDENTIFYING CORRECTLY STATED NURSING DIAGNOSES
Instructions

For the nursing diagnoses listed below, identify those correctly stated (see Appendix A when comparing). NANDA nursing diagnoses should be used for this exercise. For items inaccurately stated, amend using appropriate terminology in the space provided.

1. _____ Skin Integrity, Altered _____
2. _____ Constipation, Perceived _____
3. _____ Fluid Volume, Impaired _____
4. _____ Airway, Obstructed _____
5. _____ Fatigue _____
6. _____ Growth, Risk for Altered _____
7. _____ Confusion, Acute _____
8. _____ Incontinence, Urinary and Bowel _____
9. _____ Tissue Perfusion, Impaired _____
10. _____ Pneumonia, Risk for _____
11. _____ Hypothermia, Risk for _____
12. _____ Pain, Chronic _____
13. _____ Airway, Compromised _____
14. _____ Body Temperature, Impaired _____
15. _____ Infection, Risk for _____
16. _____ Infection, Wound _____
17. _____ Breastfeeding, Ineffective _____
18. _____ Thermoregulation, Altered _____
19. _____ Role Performance, Impaired _____
20. _____ Syndrome, Crohn's _____
21. _____ Communication, Altered Verbal _____
22. _____ Abdominal Pain _____
23. _____ Coping, Ineffective _____
24. _____ Self-Concept, Enhanced _____
25. _____ Parenting, Risk for Impaired _____
26. _____ Role Strain, Risk for Caregiver _____
27. _____ Family Processes: Alcoholism, Ineffective _____
28. _____ Coping, Defensive _____
29. _____ Injury, Risk for _____
30. _____ Grieving, Anticipatory _____
31. _____ Body Image, Impaired Perceptual _____
32. _____ Anemia, Risk for _____
33. _____ Knowledge Impairment _____
34. _____ Violence, Risk for _____
35. _____ Urinary Incontinence, Urge _____
36. _____ Anxiety _____
37. _____ Lung Cancer _____
38. _____ Stress, Acute _____
39. _____ Fear _____
40. _____ Cardiac Output, Decreased _____

STUDENT PRACTICE: PRACTICING STEP ONE AND STEP TWO OF THE NURSING PROCESS

Instructions

A. *Underline* abnormal signs and symptoms (do not underline complete sentences).

B. Above abnormal data, write O, if objective data and S, if subjective data.

C. Cluster data into related groups to identify and support each problem.

D. Label actual and risk problems using NANDA nursing diagnoses (include related to, as evidenced by, or risk factors, as appropriate).

General Information

Name: Mr. C. Gonzales

Age: 68 years   **Sex:** Male   **Race:** Hispanic

Admitting Weight: 170 pounds; 78 kilograms   **Height:** 68 inches

Vital Signs: Blood pressure 148/92; respirations 22 per minute; pulse 98 per minute; temperature 97.6°F

Client's Perception of Reason for Admission: short of breath

Allergies: no known allergies (NKA)

Current Medications: enalapril (Vasotec) 5 mg BID (twice daily); hydrochlorothiazide (HCTZ) 12.5 mg qd (daily)

Admitting Medical Diagnosis: Congestive heart failure

Previous Medical History: Coronary artery disease (CAD), congestive heart failure, hypertension

Family History: Married for 37 years with two grown children and several grandchildren

Social History: Retired from railroad seven years ago; attends church services weekly; enjoys reading and flying fuel-powered model airplanes

Assessment Data

Oxygenation: Reports difficulty breathing and increased fatigue; sleeps sitting up in recliner, other wise, unable to breathe. States he is a nonsmoker. Lung sounds with crackles to bilateral lower lung fields, anterior and posterior; non-productive cough. Apical pulse 98, strong and regular; radial pulses are equal in strength and quality. Pedal pulses are regular and equal in strength. Denies chest pain. Brisk capillary refill of fingernail beds. Pitting edema assessed to bilateral ankles and feet, rated as two-plus.

Temperature: Afebrile

Nutritional/Fluid: Saline lock inserted in right hand; patent and without erythema (redness) or edema. Reports recent weight gain of eight pounds over previous two weeks. Eats three small meals daily and drinks adequate fluids; no nausea or vomiting.

Gastrointestinal/Elimination: Reports regular bowel movement and urinary elimination patterns. Abdomen is slightly distended, soft, and non-tender to palpation. Bowel sounds are present in all four quadrants.

Rest/Sleep: States no energy and is not resting at night. Over previous two weeks has had to sleep slightly elevated in his recliner chair or becomes too short of breath. Denies use of sleeping aids or medications.

Pain Avoidance: Denies pain at this time.

Sexuality/Reproduction: Denies difficulties.

Activity: Ambulates without difficulty, however becomes short of breath with minimal exertion. States he walks around the block twice weekly.
Additional Data: Patient is alert and oriented; responds appropriately to questions.

Separate data into subjective and objective.

Subjective	Objective

Cluster data into groups of related data to determine problems.

_____

_____

_____

_____

_____

_____

_____

Determine NANDA nursing diagnosis.

_____

_____

_____

_____

_____

_____

_____

Planning

STANDARD 3: *OUTCOMES IDENTIFICATION*

The registered nurse identifies expected outcomes for a plan individualized to the patient or the situation.

Measurement Criteria

The registered nurse:

- Involves the patient, family, and other health care providers in formulating expected outcomes when possible and appropriate.
- Derives culturally appropriate expected outcomes from the diagnoses.
- Considers associated risks, benefits, costs, current scientific evidence, and clinical expertise when formulating expected outcomes.
- Defines expected outcomes in terms of the patient, patient values, ethical considerations, environment, or situation with such consideration as associated risks, benefits and costs, and current scientific evidence.
- Includes a time estimate for attainment of expected outcomes.
- Develops expected outcomes that provide direction for continuity of care.
- Modifies expected outcomes based on changes in the status of the patient or evaluation of the situation.
- Documents expected outcomes as measurable goals.

STANDARD 4: *PLANNING*

The registered nurse develops a plan that prescribes strategies and alternatives to attain expected outcomes.

Measurement Criteria

The registered nurse:

- Develops an individualized plan considering patient characteristics or the situation (e.g., age and culturally appropriated, environmentally sensitive).
- Develops the plan in conjunction with the patient, family, and others, as appropriate.
- Includes strategies within the plan that address each of the identified diagnoses or issues, which may include strategies for promotion and restoration of health and prevention of illness, injury, and disease.
- Provides for continuity within the plan.
- Incorporates an implementation pathway or timeline within the plan.
- Establishes the plan priorities with the patient, family, and others as appropriate.
- Utilizes the plan to provide direction to other members of the health care team.
- Defines the plan to reflect current statues, rules and regulations, and standards.
- Integrates current trends and research affecting care in the planning process.
- Considers the economic impact of the plan.
- Uses standardized language or recognized terminology to document the plan.

(From American Nurses Association. [2004]. *Nursing: Scope and standards of practice*. Washington, DC: Author.)

OBJECTIVES

Upon completion of this chapter, the student should be able to:

- Define the purposes of the planning phase.
- Identify and describe each component of the planning phase.
- Distinguish between goals and expected outcomes.
- Explain characteristics of nursing interventions and rationales.
- Discuss communication and documentation of the care plan.

KEY TERMS

care plan
client centered
dependent nursing
    intervention
discharge planning
expected outcome
goal

independent nursing
    intervention
interdependent nursing
    intervention
long-term goal
measurable
nursing intervention

planning
priority
rationale
short-term goal
strengths

PLANNING: STEP 3 OF THE NURSING PROCESS

Planning is the third phase of the nursing process. In prior steps, data were collected, analyzed, validated, and organized, and problems and strengths identified, then labeled with the appropriate nursing diagnosis. Nurses then develop a plan of care, which establishes the proposed course of nursing action. The ultimate goal of the planning phase is to promote optimum or an improved level of functioning for the client. Critical elements of planning include:

- Identifying priority problems and interventions.
- Setting realistic goals and expected outcomes.
- Determining appropriate nursing interventions and recognizing when collaboration is necessary.
- Communicating and documenting the proposed care plan.

Scientific knowledge and understanding of the holistic needs of the client aid the professional nurse in effective planning. The purpose of this chapter is to explain the above critical components and to stress the importance of effective planning in promoting quality nursing care.

Planning begins as the nurse analyzes the overall data collected during the assessment phase and the client's health care situation. Critical thought and problem solving are necessary skills when planning care. *Priority* problems requiring immediate attention are identified. *Strengths*, the client's *support system*, the health care *facility* itself, and available *resources* are considered, as well.

Priority problems are those appraised to be more important or life threatening. Priorities are dealt with before less critical problems. For example, Terrence Stewart was involved in an automobile accident and arrived at an emergency care center for treatment. Mr. Stewart began to experience symptoms suspiciously similar to an acute myocardial infarction (heart attack). In addition, he had sustained abrasions (skin scrapes) to his left arm and elbow during the accident. Obviously, the priority in this scenario is providing care to support the client's circulatory system (or cardiac function). The abrasions may be recognized as a problem, but they are less critical.

Strengths include physical, psychological, or personal characteristics. Strengths are thought to *promote* a higher or improved level of functioning. Examples of strengths include:

- Physical: client has maintained optimal physical condition with exercise or diet.
- Psychological: client exhibits healthy ways of coping in a crisis.
- Personal: client is motivated to recover independence; compliance with medical treatment.

Facility refers to the health care delivery facility. The facility must be capable of providing the care necessary for a client. For example, if a client was a resident in a long-term care facility and sustained an injury requiring surgical intervention, this client will most likely require transfer to another facility equipped to provide surgical care. If another client began experiencing chest pain radiating to his left arm, and experienced nausea and shortness of breath (dyspnea), the most appropriate facility would be an acute care facility, not a health clinic.

Resources refer to the ways and means of obtaining health care. For example, is necessary equipment available at the facility? Does the client have transportation to obtain health care? Does the client have health insurance? Can the client afford to purchase medication or equipment prescribed?

Every aspect of the care plan should be *realistic* for both the client and the hospital, facility, or home care setting, depending on client needs.

Purpose and Characteristics of Planning

Planning care must be individualized and realistic for each client. The purpose of planning includes promoting improvement in the client's present state of health or preserving the client's present health status. Planning facilitates adjustment to diminished health, when an improved level of wellness is not possible, or promotes acceptance to the client's deteriorating health. Steps involved in planning include:

- Determining priority problems.
- Establishing goals and expected outcomes.
- Planing interventions with scientific rationale.
- Communicating and documenting the plan of care.

DETERMINING PRIORITIES

The first step in planning is determining **priorities** by recognizing problems that need immediate attention. Obviously, life-threatening situations must be given more urgency than non-life-threatening problems. Consider client preferences by encouraging input. Mutually setting priorities promotes compliance with care and the client's sense of control. Table 4:1 shows common guidelines to assist in priority setting.

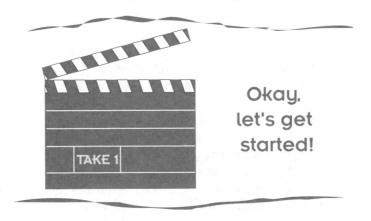

Okay, let's get started!

Consider *Maslow's hierarchy of needs*. Prioritize according to the basic physiological needs (oxygenation, nutrition, hydration, elimination, body temperature maintenance, and pain avoidance). Generally, basic

TABLE 4:1 Associating Maslow's Hierarchy of Needs with Priority Problems

Priority 1 Physiological needs	• Problems interfering with ability to maintain physiological life processes, such as ability to breathe, maintaining a patent airway, maintaining adequate circulation. • Problems interfering with homeostatic physiological responses within the body, such as respiration, circulation, hydration, elimination, temperature regulation, nutrition. • Problems interfering with ability to be free of offensive stimuli, such as pain, nausea, and other physical irritation.
Priority 2 Safety/security	• Problems interfering with safety and security, such as anxiety, fear, environmental hazards, physical activity deficit, violence towards self or others.
Priority 3 Love and belonging	• Problems interfering with love and belonging, such as sensory-perceptual losses, inability to maintain family and significant other relationships, isolation, loss of a loved one.
Priority 4 Self-esteem	• Problems interfering with self-esteem, such as inability to perform normal daily activities of living, change in physiological structure or function of body or body part.
Priority 5 Self-actualization	• Problems interfering with one's ability for self-actualization, such as positive personal assessment of life events, achieving personal goals.

physiological needs must be met sufficiently, before higher level needs (safe environment, security, love and belonging, and so on) are addressed.

Attention to more than one problem may occur simultaneously. For example, the nurse may be performing interventions related to pain reduction and, at the same time, instructing and encouraging

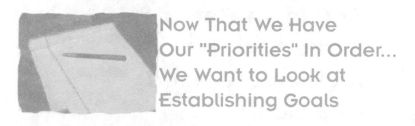

Now That We Have Our "Priorities" In Order... We Want to Look at Establishing Goals

TABLE 4:2 Prioritizing Nursing Diagnoses with Accompanying Nursing Interventions

Priority	Nursing Diagnosis	Nursing Interventions
High	Risk for suffocation	• Encourage safety measures • Maintain proper positioning • Suction as needed
Moderate	Risk for impaired skin integrity	• Perform comprehensive skin assessment • Keep skin clean and dry • Provide turning schedule
Low	Ineffective coping	• Assist to identify problems • Encourage keeping daily journal • Teach client strategies for expressing feelings

the client about proper use of an incentive spirometer, thus improving the client's oxygenation status.

Finally, priorities may include setting goals and instituting actions to prevent problems from occurring (see Table 4:2). Nurses often anticipate potentially serious problems that may arise without nursing intervention.

Goals and expected outcomes:

• Give direction to the plan of care.
• Are used to evaluate the effectiveness of the nursing care plan.

ESTABLISHING GOALS AND EXPECTED OUTCOMES

After priority problem identification, setting goals and expected outcomes follows. One overall goal is determined for each nursing diagnosis.

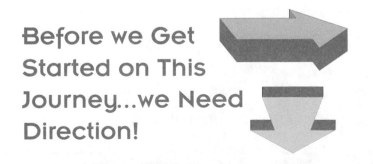

Before we Get Started on This Journey...we Need Direction!

Table 4:3 Application of Goals and Expected Outcomes

Nursing Diagnosis: *Body image disturbed*

Goal: Client will demonstrate acceptance of amputation and an ability to adjust to lifestyle change within six months.

Expected Outcomes:
- Looks at and touches area of missing body part
- Participates in wound/stump care
- Plans for prosthesis
- Returns to former social involvement

Nursing Diagnosis: *Impaired gas exchange*

Goal: Client will maintain a patent airway throughout hospitalization.

Expected Outcomes:
- Verbalizes understanding of oxygen administration and respiratory treatments
- Maintains adequate oxygenation and ventilation
- Remains free of signs of respiratory distress

Definition and Components of Goals and Expected Outcomes

The terms *goal, outcome,* and *expected outcome* are often used interchangeably. A goal is a general statement indicating the intent or desired change in the client's health status, function, or behavior. An expected outcome is more specific, describing the methods through which the goal will be achieved. Refer to Table 4:3 for goal and expected outcome application examples.

Goals and expected outcomes must be measurable (able to be quantified). The client demonstrates a certain action within a specified time frame. The demonstrated action and time frame are the yardsticks which allow the goal or expected outcome to be measured. As interventions planned with goal resolution in mind are carried out, nurses determine how the client responds to each intervention. Favorable responses will most likely lead to attainment of goals and resolution of problems. Goals and expected outcomes provide the health care team with a clear understanding of what is to be accomplished. Goals and expected outcomes are client centered. The client (or part of the client) is expected to achieve a desired outcome.

Goals are constructed by focusing on problem prevention, resolution, and/or rehabilitation. A short-term goal is a statement identifying a change in behavior that can be achieved fairly quickly, usually within a few hours or days. A long-term goal indicates an objective to be achieved over a longer period, usually over weeks or months. Long-term goals focus on overall greater expectations that may require ongoing health care attention. Discharge planning involves identifying long-term goals, thus promoting continued restorative care and problem resolution through home health, physical therapy, or various other referral sources (Figure 4:1).

After the goal is stated, expected outcomes are identified. Expected outcomes are measurable steps indicating progress toward goal achievement. For each nursing diagnosis and overall goal, there may be

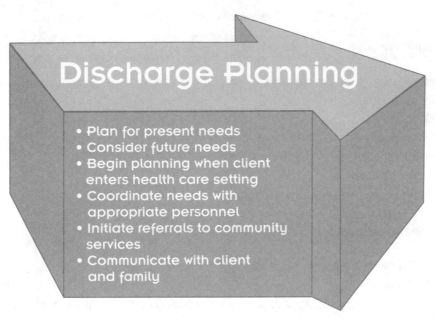

FIGURE 4:1 Goals for Discharge Planning.

several expected outcomes. Both goals and expected outcomes include specific components when appropriately expressed (see Table 4:4 for examples of common mistakes in writing goals). Components include: subject, behavior, performance criteria, and time frame.

- The subject identifies the person who will perform the desired behavior or meet the goal. Since goals are client centered, subject refers to the client.
- Behavior describes *what* the client will do to achieve the goal (see Table 4:5 for examples of measurable verbs). Behavior can be felt, heard, seen, or measured. For example:
  - Will verbalize
  - Will ambulate
  - Will report
  - Will eat
  - Will demonstrate
- The criteria of performance refer to the standards indicating the level of behavior, such as how long, how far, how much. Criteria of performance may include a time limit, amount of activity, or description of the behavior to be followed.

Examples include:

- Understanding of medication regime
- Length of the hall
- Decrease in pain level of four or less
- Seventy-five percent of meal
- Decreased blood pressure within 48 hours

TABLE 4:4 Common Mistakes in Writing Goals

Incorrect	Correct
• Focus on the nurse's action when writing the goal	• Goals must be client centered. The *subject* in the goal is the client. For example, *client will demonstrate correct self-administration technique of insulin injection within forty-eight hours of initial instruction.*
• Statement of unrealistic goal for client. For example, a client with advanced Alzheimer's, incontinent of urine, whose care plan goal reads: client will remain continent throughout hospitalization.	• Goals should be realistic. Ask yourself, can the client perform the stated action, thus achieving the goal within the stated time frame? For the incontinent client with advanced Alzheimer's, a more appropriate goal might be stated: *client will maintain skin integrity as evidenced by use of continence aids to keep skin dry throughout shift.*
• Goal lacks time frame	• The time frame indicates *when* the goal should be achieved. Otherwise, determination of the client's success or failure in achieving the desired result can not be evaluated. Appropriately stated goals require four components: subject (*the client*), behavior (*will maintain*), criteria of performance (*skin integrity*), and time frame (*throughout shift*). A fifth component, conditions, is optional. In the example above, *use of continence aids to keep skin dry,* is the condition.
• More than one task or behavior to be accomplished in one goal statement. For example, client will demonstrate a tolerable level of discomfort and will identify at least two alternative measures to reduce pain level within eight hours.	• Only one behavior should be specified for each goal. Goals will be more explicit and directly measurable.

• Conditions, *an optional component,* refer to the aid or conditions which facilitate the performance. Conditions may provide clarity. They include experiences the client is expected to have before performing the behavior. For example:
  • With the assistance of physical therapy
  • With the administration of analgesics

TABLE 4:5 Measurable Verbs

Identify	Describe	Perform	Relate
State	List	Verbalize	Hold
Demonstrate	Share	Express	Sit
Exercise	Communicate	Stand	Discuss
Cough	Walk	Describe	Reestablish

- With assistance of family
- With use of medication and diet therapy
- The time frame refers to when the behavior should be accomplished. For example:
  - Within 48 hours
  - By third postoperative day
  - Within 45 minutes
  - In 24 hours
  - Within three weeks of medication therapy

WRITING GOAL AND OUTCOME STATEMENTS

The following are examples of goals stated correctly:

- Client will ambulate assisted by physical therapy to nurse's station and back to room twice daily.
- Client will verbalize understanding of medication regime prior to discharge.
- Client's skin will demonstrate no evidence of breakdown throughout hospitalization.
- Ms. James will lose two-and-a-half lbs. within three weeks by using prescribed American Heart Association Diet plan.
- Client will ambulate unassisted with crutches by discharge.
- Client will demonstrate correct injection technique by September 18.

Nursing Intervention Classification (NIC) and Nursing Outcomes Classification (NOC) Defined

The University of Iowa (Iowa Intervention Project) developed the nomenclature of nursing interventions known as *Nursing Interventions Classifications* (NIC), directed towards health promotion and illness management. NIC continues to refine the standardized language that describes nursing interventions performed in all practice settings. NIC is a method for linking nursing interventions to diagnoses and client outcomes. Each intervention is labeled, defined, and lists activities the nurse performs while carrying out the intervention (University of Iowa [n.d.]).

With nursing communities placing greater interest on nursing outcomes, nurse researchers at the University of Iowa have further developed classifications, *Nursing Outcomes Classification* (NOC), of client outcomes. According to the University of Iowa, an outcome is a measurable individual, family or community state, behavior or perception that is measured along a continuum and is responsive to nursing interventions. NOC continues to be refined for measuring effects of nursing practice.

Nursing researchers are involved in observing, measuring, and studying client outcomes which indicate the quality of effectiveness on the nursing interventions provided. The 330 outcomes are grouped into 31 classes and seven domains for ease of use.

STUDENT PRACTICE: WRITING GOALS
Instructions

For each nursing diagnosis write an appropriate goal. (Remember goal components.)

1. Joe Johnson has experienced intermittent nausea for approximately six months due to a possible gastric ulcer. He states, "I know I should eat, but when I eat, I hurt." He has lost 28 pounds since his last annual checkup and weighs less than is ideal for his height. His nurse identifies the nursing diagnosis: *Imbalanced Nutrition: Less than Body Requirements*; R/T: inability to ingest nutrients as a result of biological factors; AEB: reported food intake less than recommended daily allowance; weight loss of 28 pounds over last year.

_____

_____

2. Hannah Miller, a neonate, is experiencing a fluctuation in her body temperature from normal to below normal range. Her nurse discovers that Hannah's mother does not keep her covered appropriately. The nurse identifies the nursing diagnosis: *Risk for Hypothermia*; risk factors: exposure to cool environment, inadequate clothing, extremes of age (newborn).

_____

_____

3. Mr. Cooper had abdominal surgery one day ago. He has a medical history of diabetes mellitus and must take morning and evening insulin subcutaneously. His nurse identifies the nursing diagnosis: *Risk for Infection*; R/T: inadequate primary defenses (surgical incision/broken skin), increased environmental exposure, chronic disease, invasive procedures.

_____

_____

4. Mr. Sanders states he has been traveling out of the country. Since his return last week, he has been experiencing abdominal cramping and several liquid stools. The nursing diagnosis identified is *Diarrhea*; R/T: gastrointestinal disorder; AEB: abdominal cramping, increased frequency of defecation, liquid stools.

_____

_____

5. Mrs. O'Conner was admitted to the hospital diagnosed with pneumonia. Assessment reveals bilateral wheezes in the midanterior lung fields and mild dyspnea. The nurse observes Mrs. O'Conner coughing up copious amounts of thick, yellow sputum. The nursing diagnosis is identified as *Ineffective*

Airway Clearance; R/T: tracheobronchial infection; AEB: abnormal breath sounds (wheezes), productive cough, dyspnea.

Nursing Tip

Planning is
One . . . Identifying Priorities
Two . . . Setting Goals
And
Three . . . Planning Nursing Interventions

PLANNING NURSING INTERVENTIONS

After prioritizing problems and setting goals, nurses use problem-solving and decision-making skills in determining what actions will aid in problem resolution. **Nursing interventions** are specified activities executed by the nursing team which benefit the client in a predictable manner.

Nursing Tip

Interventions are actions carried out
by nurses to meet goals and,
therefore, to resolve identified
actual or potential problems.

Characteristics of Nursing Interventions

Nursing interventions are activities or actions planned by the nurse to produce problem resolution, problem reduction, or prevention of risk problems. Nursing interventions may be planned to assist the client accept his or her present state of health or illness. Nursing interventions specify activities to execute.

They focus on the etiology of the problem and may determine when activities are to be carried out, how often, and the duration for each activity.

Nursing interventions are communicated to other nurses involved in the client's treatment by verbal or written report and through documentation of the plan, which promotes continuity of care.

Nursing Tip

Nursing interventions involve:

- Assisting with activities of daily living (ADLs)
- Delivering skilled therapeutic interventions
- Discharge planning

- Monitoring response to medical and nursing care
- Supervising and coordinating nursing personnel
- Teaching the client

Guidelines for Selecting Nursing Interventions

Appropriate interventions are selected using guiding principles provided by official nurse regulating organizations, such as individual nurse practice acts, state boards of nursing standards, and the JCAHO standards for nursing care. Nurses must practice within the legal realm of nursing guidelines and boundaries. Furthermore, interventions must be realistic for the client and nurse, as well as for the facility. Nurses consider the client's values and beliefs and the consequences and risks of each intervention.

Classification of Nursing Interventions

Nursing interventions are classified according to three categories:

- Independent
- Interdependent
- Dependent

Independent nursing interventions are nursing actions initiated by the nurse not requiring direction or an order from another health care professional. They are actions regulated by state boards of nursing and nurse practice acts, which allow nurses to independently intervene depending on client needs. Interventions may support ADLs, health education, health promotion, and counseling. For example, the environment may be managed by nurses to establish and maintain a safe, therapeutic environment, promote rest, reduce noise, maintain cleanliness, or manage environmental temperature.

Interdependent nursing interventions are actions developed in consultation or collaboration with other health care professionals to gain another's viewpoint in determining an intervention most beneficial for the client. An example would be discussion of the client in an interdisciplinary conference for discharge planning, attended by the primary nurse or supervisor, home health care nurse, social worker, physical therapist, and dietician.

Nurses may consult with specialists when the problem cannot be resolved using their personal knowledge or skills. Specialists may be consulted to determine the best method for nursing diagnosis resolution, for example, consulting a dietician regarding a special diet.

Dependent nursing interventions are actions requiring an order from a physician or another health care professional, such as a request for physician-prescribed medication orders. Likewise, nurses may question a previously written order based on knowledge of current client status or change in the client's condition, requesting clarification or new orders.

Where Do Nursing Interventions Originate?

Interventions may originate from written or verbal physician orders. The physician relies on the nurse's judgment and ability to carry out orders in a safe, effective manner. Nursing interventions may be written to complement the physician-prescribed treatments (see Table 4:6).

Nursing interventions may result from such client needs as health-related teaching, counseling, or referrals to other health care professionals. Interventions may involve specific nursing treatments or collection of ongoing assessment data related to client status. Other interventions may evolve from measures to take during basic care, such as suctioning, repositioning, assisting with nutrition, providing hygiene measures, assisting with ADLs, providing emotional support, or maintaining range of motion.

Example:
Nursing diagnosis: *Activity intolerance*; R/T: bed rest, generalized weakness; AEB: verbalization of overwhelming lack of energy, dyspnea on exertion while performing activities of daily living.
Goal: *Client will verbalize improved level of energy when carrying out activities of daily living within one week.*

1. Assess ability to perform ADLs.
2. Evaluate adequacy of nutrition and sleep.
3. Schedule periods of uninterrupted time for client to rest throughout the day.
4. Assist client with activities of daily living as necessary. Promote and encourage ADL independence without causing exhaustion.

Interventions are prioritized according to the order in which they will be implemented or carried out. Several interventions should be identified for each goal.

Scientific Rationales

As previously explained, interventions are selected based on an understanding of scientific principles and psychosocial or developmental theories. Understanding of the human body and mind allows for certain expected responses when interventions are carried out. Rationales are the underlying reasons for which the intervention was chosen. When interventions are chosen, nursing students should identify and provide scientific rationale for each intervention. This action aids in further understanding of the theoretical and scientific knowledge of nursing.

Example:
The nurse is caring for a client medically diagnosed with emphysema who refuses to quit smoking cigarettes.

TABLE 4:6 Types of Nursing Orders

Type	Description	Example
Health Promotion	Encouraging behaviors leading to a higher level of wellness	• Reinforce the importance of a daily exercise regimen. • Encourage client to begin keeping a journal of daily exercises performed.
Observation/Monitoring Patient Status	Monitoring client for potential complications and response to performed nursing interventions	• Encourage client to report increasing pain level prior to it becoming severe • Monitor blood pressure prior to administering antihypertensive medications as ordered by provider
Prevention	Reducing risk factors or preventing complications	• Encourage client to use incentive spirometer every two hours and monitor performance • Advise client and family members in proper handwashing method
Treatment	Teaching, referrals, or performing physical care necessary in the treatment of an existing problem	• Teach client proper technique for diabetic foot care • Request referral for dietary consult

Nursing diagnosis: *Noncompliance* (therapeutic regime)
R/T: client value system, health belief
AEB: failure to adhere to health recommendations, evidence of exacerbation of symptoms
Goal: *Client will communicate an understanding of disease process and treatment within 48 hours.*
Nursing Intervention: Collaborate with client to implement a plan for smoking cessation.
Rationale: *Active participation in decision making about therapeutic regime may increase compliance.*

Scientific research has provided proof that a client who participates in health care decision making is more likely to be compliant. This data may be located in research articles, fundamental or foundation

Nursing Tip

Determine key words in interventions and diagnoses, such as postsurgery and hypoxia. Rationales for these would be found in medical-surgical textbook chapters relating to any client undergoing surgery for any reason. Hypoxia is a postoperative complication for which the nurse must monitor.

textbooks, nursing journals, and other resources. Identify the *key subject* or *term*, such as decision making or compliance, and then locate the rationale in one of the resources or references.

Example:
For the client who had orthopedic surgery:
Nursing intervention: Monitor airway and respiratory pattern every two hours for initial eight to twelve hours or until stable.
Rationale: *Most anesthetic agents depress respiratory rate and depth, thus interfering with oxygenation of the blood.*

Side effects and adverse effects of anesthetic agents are found in resources, such as medical-surgical textbooks discussing the care of surgical clients.

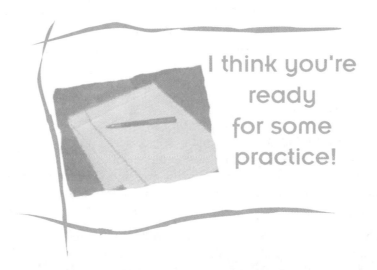

I think you're ready for some practice!

STUDENT PRACTICE: SCIENTIFIC RATIONALES

Instructions

Determine scientific rationales for each nursing intervention below.

Nursing diagnosis: *Activity intolerance*; R/T: bed rest, generalized weakness; AEB: verbalization of overwhelming lack of energy, dyspnea on exertion while performing ADLs

Goal: *Client will verbalize improved level of energy when carrying out ADLs within one week.*

Nursing Interventions:

1. Assess ability to perform activities of daily living. _____

   _____

   _____

2. Determine cause of activity intolerance and determine if the cause is physical or motivational.

   _____

   _____

3. Encourage client to be out of bed. Increase activity gradually. _____

   _____

   _____

4. Allow clients sufficient time to carry out activities of daily living and give adequate rest periods between activities. Provide assistance as necessary.

   _____

   _____

COMMUNICATING AND DOCUMENTING THE CARE PLAN

The client's plan of care is documented according to hospital policy and becomes part of the client's permanent medical record. The care plan is shared with other members of the health care team who are actively caring for the client. The plan may be reviewed by the oncoming nurse or communicated in part during report.

KEY CONCEPTS

- Planning is the third phase in the nursing process. Critical elements of planning include identifying priority problems and interventions, setting realistic goals and expected outcomes, determining nursing interventions and rationales for each intervention, and finally, communication and documentation of the care plan.

- Establishing priorities may be guided by factors such as endangerment to life, client preferences, and Maslow's hierarchy of needs.
- The care plan is realistic and practical. It considers the client's values, beliefs, and strengths, as well as physical and psychological health.
- Planning individualized care for the client may promote improvement of health, preserve the client's present state of health, help the client to adjust to diminished or a decreasing level of health, or assist the client in accepting deteriorating health.
- A goal indicates the desired change in the client's health status. Goals are client centered and give direction to the care plan. Goals are constructed by focusing on problem prevention, resolution, or rehabilitation. Components of a goal statement include the subject, behavior, criteria of performance, conditions, and time frame.
- Expected outcomes are more specific than goals and describe the methods through which the goal is achieved.
- Goals and expected outcomes are used to measure the success of the care plan. Goals and expected outcomes are stated in a manner that makes them measurable.
- Nursing interventions are actions to be carried out by the nurse and are expected to benefit the client in a predictable manner. Interventions are developed to meet goal objectives and therefore aid in problem resolution.
- Nursing interventions are selected based on the nurse's understanding of scientific principles and psychological or developmental theories. Rationales are the underlying scientific reason for which the intervention was chosen.
- The nursing care plan is a formal written document that becomes part of the client's permanent medical record.
- Documentation and communication of the plan promotes continuity of care.

STUDENT PRACTICE: PLANNING AND OUTCOME IDENTIFICATION
Instructions

Using the scenario from Chapter 3, Mr. C. Gonzales, whose medical diagnosis is congestive heart failure (CHF):

1. Complete all steps involved in planning and outcome identification. (See chart, Figure 4:2.)
2. Identify two or three priority problems. For each problem, determine one nursing diagnosis statement (label, R/T, and AEB), one goal, and three interventions with scientific rationale.

Name: _____ Date: _____

Care plan documentation form: For each nursing diagnosis, include R/T, AEB, or risk factors (for risk nursing diagnosis); one goal/expected outcome per nursing diagnosis; and at least three nursing interventions with scientific rationale for each nursing intervention. Evaluate goal/expected outcome when appropriate (one evaluative statement).

Nursing Diagnosis (with R/T + AEB)

_____

_____

Goal

_____

_____

Nursing Interventions (with *Scientific Rationale*)

1 _____

_____

_____

2. _____

_____

_____

3. _____

_____

_____

Evaluation

_____

_____

FIGURE 4:2 Care Plan Documentation Form.

Implementation

STANDARD 5: *IMPLEMENTATION*

The registered nurse implements the identified plan.

Measurement Criteria

The registered nurse:

- Implements the plan in a safe and timely manner.
- Documents implementation and any modification, including changes or omissions, of the identified plan.
- Utilizes evidence-based interventions and treatments specific to the diagnosis or problem.
- Utilizes community resources and systems to implement the plan.
- Collaborates with nursing colleagues and others to implement the plan.

STANDARD 5A: *COORDINATION OF CARE*

The registered nurse coordinates care delivery.

Measurement Criteria

The registered nurse:

- Coordinates implementation of the plan.
- Documents the coordination of the care.

STANDARD 5B: *HEALTH TEACHING AND HEALTH PROMOTION*

The registered nurse employs strategies to promote health and a safe environment.

Measurement Criteria

The registered nurse:

- Provides health teaching that addresses such topics as health lifestyles, risk-reducing behaviors, developmental needs, activities of daily living, and preventive self-care.
- Uses health promotion and health teaching methods appropriate to the situation and the patient's developmental level, learning needs, readiness, ability to learn, language preference, and culture.
- Seeks opportunities for feedback and evaluation of the effectiveness of the strategies used.

(From American Nurses Association. [2004]. *Nursing: Scope and standards of practice*. Washington, DC: Author).

OBJECTIVES

Upon completion of this chapter, the student should be able to:

- Discuss the purpose of the implementation phase of the nursing process.
- Describe ways in which the care plan is implemented.
- Identify the relationship between assessment and implementation.
- Discuss communication and documentation of client response to interventions as they are implemented.

- Describe key components of recording and reporting, including data to document on the client's chart and data to report to oncoming personnel.
- Discuss confidentiality and the client's right to privacy.

KEY TERMS

confidentiality
documentation
focus charting

implementation
Kardex
narrative charting

PIE charting
reporting

IMPLEMENTATION: STEP 4 OF THE NURSING PROCESS

Implementation is the fourth phase of the nursing process. During this phase, activities such as executing nursing interventions, performing an ongoing assessment of the client, and determining the client's response to executed interventions are observed, communicated, and documented. As with all prior steps of the nursing process, nurses demonstrate knowledge and understanding of physical and social sciences and apply analytical skills and deliberate thought processes to interpret client responses to interventions. Nurses participate in ongoing assessment as implementation takes place. This chapter discusses the purpose and characteristics of implementation, guidelines for reporting and recording, and the client's right to privacy and confidentiality.

Characteristics of Implementation

The implementation phase is directed at meeting the client's needs through execution of interventions and evaluation of client response. These actions ultimately result in health promotion, prevention of illness, or restoration of health. The client is encouraged to provide input in care planning and priority identification, thus promoting compliance and giving the client a sense of control.

Nursing professionals monitor the client's response to treatment and therapies through means of physical assessment and communication with the client. Nurses analyze the client's response. Evaluation may include additional inquiry, such as reviewing laboratory results, progress notes, and collaborating with the physician and other nurses involved in the client's care. Accurate reporting and recording of all pertinent data are necessary.

DOCUMENTATION

Several factors are considered for documentation to be effective. Documentation is the process of preparing a record reflecting the assessment data and both the client's health status and response to care. Depending on the facility, various formats may be used. Guidelines for documentation include the following:

- Ensure that you have the correct client record or chart and that the client's name and identifying information are on every page of the record.

CHAPTER FIVE

- Document as soon as the client encounter is concluded to ensure accurate recall of data (follow institutional guidelines on frequency of charting).
- Date and time each entry.
- Sign each entry with your full legal name and with your professional credentials, or per your institutional policy.
- Do not leave space between entries.
- If an error is made while documenting, use a single line to cross out the error, then date, time, and sign the correction (check institutional policy); avoid erasing, crossing out, or using correction fluid.
- Never change another person's entry, even if it is incorrect.
- Use quotation marks to indicate direct client responses (e.g., "I feel lousy").
- Document in chronological order (if chronological order is not used, state why).
- Write legibly.
- Use a permanent ink pen (black is usually preferable because of its ability to photocopy well).
- Document in a complete but concise manner by using phrases and abbreviations as appropriate.
- Document all telephone calls that you make or receive that are related to a client's case.

(Adapted from Estes, M.E.Z. [2002]. *Health assessment and physical examination* [2nd ed.]. Albany, NY: Thomson Delmar Learning.)

Assessment Specific Documentation Guidelines

- Record all data that contribute directly to the assessment (e.g., positive assessment findings and pertinent negatives).
- Document any parts of the assessment that are omitted or refused by the client.
- Avoid using judgmental language such as "good," "poor," "bad," "normal," "abnormal," "decreased," "appears to be," and "seems."
- Avoid evaluative statements (e.g., "client is uncooperative," "client is lazy"); cite instead specific statements or actions that you observe (e.g., "client said 'I hate this place' and kicked trash can").
- State time intervals precisely (e.g., "every four hours," "bid," instead of seldom," "occasionally").
- Do not make relative statements about findings (e.g., "mass the size of an egg"); use specific measurements (e.g., "mass 3 cm x 5 cm").
- Draw pictures when appropriate (e.g., location of scar, masses, skin lesion, decubitus, deep tendon reflex, etc.).
- Refer to findings using anatomical landmarks (e.g., left upper quadrant [of abdomen], left lower lobe [of lung], midclavicular line, etc.).
- Use the face of the clock to describe findings that are in a circular pattern (e.g., breast, tympanic membrane, rectum, vagina).
- Document any change in the client's condition during a visit or from previous visits.
- Describe what you observed, not what you did.

(Adapted from Estes, M.E.Z. [2002]. *Health assessment and physical examination* [2nd ed.]. Albany, NY: Thomson Delmar Learning.)

Figure 5:1 compares examples of correctly and incorrectly documented data on a 24-hour record.

SEE CARE PLAN
NURSING DIAGNOSIS

Do not leave blank lines between entries.

Write legibly. Sign each entry with name and credentials.

Date	Time	Progress Notes
X/XX/XX	0840	AM ~~~ completed by nurses aid.-------- Cmnussi
	0930	16F Foley cath inserted, s que. 450cc clear yellow urine out.
	1100	Husband at bedside. Seems to be mad at wife. J.Minton RN
	1340	Pt. To x-ray via ~~stretcher~~ wheelchair.

Don't leave blank spaces after entry.

When an error is made, draw one line through entry. Write 'incorrect entry' and initial.

SEE CARE PLAN
NURSING DIAGNOSIS:

Date	Time	Progress Notes
X/XX/XX	0700	Received pt. Sitting on bedside chair. Respirations, even, un-labored. Skin warm, dry. No distress noted.—J.Minton RN
	0845	Breakfast served, family at bedside. Denies dyspnea or____ chest pain at this time, however, using ~~assessory muscles~~ *incorrect entry – JM* accessory muscles to breath, at rest.---- J. Minton RN

FIGURE 5:1 Examples of Incorrect and Correct Documentation.

Nursing Tip

Effective documentation requires:
- Use of a common vocabulary
- Legibility and neatness
- Use of only authorized abbreviations and symbols
- Factual and time-sequenced organization
- Accurately including any errors that occurred
- Following facility protocol

Documentation Methods

Depending on your facility, many different systems may be utilized for documentation purposes: narrative, PIE, focus, and others. Always be familiar with your facility's documentation policies and procedures, and document within those guidelines.

Narrative Charting

Narrative charting refers to a traditional, sequential, documentation system. The nurse describes the client's status, physical assessment, interventions and treatments, and the client's response to treatments. Narrative charting has been replaced in many institutions because:

- The flow of care is disorganized.
- It fails to reflect the nursing process.
- It is time consuming.
- Specific information is difficult to retrieve.

Be specific and descriptive when documenting narrative notes. See the acronym CHARTING in Table 5:1 for data to include.

PIE Charting

PIE (problem-intervention-evaluation) charting organizes information according to problems the client is experiencing, interventions performed, and evaluation of client response. Assessment flow sheets and progress notes are maintained on a daily basis. Initial assessment determines problems, labels them as nursing diagnoses, and numbers them for future reference. For example, when the nurse documents data regarding problem one, the entry notation begins with *P #1*. For interventions performed in relation to problem one, the entry notation begins with *I-P #1*, followed by the entry. When the nurse

TABLE 5:1 Documentation to Include While Charting

Condition: current condition of the client, physically, emotionally; condition of wounds/dressings; change in condition of client.

Happenings: abnormal or variations from usual routine; visits from family, physician, discharge instructions.

Additions: changes to the care plan; abnormal laboratory values.

Response: to interventions carried out, reactions or response to medications administered, reports received or given to other personnel.

Treatments, transfers, transport to other departments.

Invasive procedures performed.

Notes: refers to narrative notes when the flow sheet is not enough.

Good job!

SEE CARE PLAN
NURSING DIAGNOSIS:

DATE	TIME	NOTES
12/15/04	1330	P#1 = Complaints of acute pain to right lower quadrant
		abdomen. Rates as "7" on scale of 1 to 10.
		I P#1 = adm. Analgesics as prescribed. Monitor quality,
		location, intensity, & frequency. Document. Encourage
		diversional activities, such as, music, focus breathing
		reading, etc. Advise to request analgesic prior to pain
		Becoming intense------------------------W.Seaback RN
		EP#1 = pain resolves. Client requests analgesics when
		pain level "4" or less on scale of 1 to 10. Participates
		in diversional activities. VS remain within normal limits.
		Client reports further symptoms._____ W.Seaback RN
12/13/04	1330	P#2 = Risk for Infection RT surgical incision
		I P#2 = sterile wound care qd, as per MD orders.
		Monitor wound for signs of redness, edema, drainage,
		odor, approximation. Monitor for temp elevation. Adm.
		Antibiotics as ordered.------------------W.Seaback RN
		EP#2 = incision heals without evidence of infection. No
		temp elevation.------------------------W.Seaback RN

FIGURE 5:2 PIE Charting Example.

evaluates the response to an intervention for problem one, the entry notation begins with *E-P #1*, followed by the evaluation entry, and so on. Figure 5:2 shows an example of PIE documentation.

FOCUS Charting

The focus charting system involves documentation of three categories: *data*, *action*, and *response*, or DAR. Figure 5:3 shows an example of a focus charting system. The *D* or data category is the focus of the entry. Each focus may include specific identified problems stated as nursing diagnoses or may identify the topic of the entry. Examples of data may include:

- a nursing diagnosis, such as *Impaired Mobility*.
- subjective or objective data, such as description of a wound or abdominal pain.
- client behavior, such as ability to perform ADL's.
- change in the client's condition, such as labored respiration or experiencing chest pain.
- a significant event, such as debridement of a wound.
- a special need, such as referral to home health care service.

The A or *action* category includes nursing actions based on assessment of the client's condition. An example is administering an analgesic in response to the client's subjective statement of severe pain. The action entry includes the executed intervention. Actions may also include changes to the care plan deemed necessary, resulting from the nurse's assessment.

SEE CARE PLAN
NURSING DIAGNOSIS:

Date	Time	Focus	Progress Notes
5/3/04	0945	Consti-	D: Pt states no BM for 4 days. Abdominal
		pation	cramping. Bowel sounds hypoactive X 4 quads
	1015		A: administered 1000 cc warm, tap-water
			enema. Advised to hold as long as possible.
	1055		A: assisted to bedside commode. Call bell
			within reach.----------------W.Seaback RN
	1100		R: Client expelled large amount of dark,
			brown, formed stool, large amount of liquid
			and flatus.-------------- W.Seaback RN
	1130		A: assisted into bed. Provided perineal care.
			D: excoriation noted to perineal area. Skin
			barrier applied. ------------W.Seaback RN
	1300	Nutri-	D: client ate 75% of soft mechanical diet.
		tion	No nausea at this time.------W.Seaback RN

FIGURE 5:3 FOCUS Charting Example.

The *response* category (R) describes the client's response to nursing care, medical care, or specific interventions. In the example of administering an analgesic for severe pain, the response entry might include a statement noting severe pain was resolved.

Computerized Documentation

Many health care organizations have implemented computerized documentation in response to the large demand for clinical, administrative, and regulatory information. Health care facilities work in collaboration with producers of computer software to design medical record documents that complement existing documentation systems. There are advantages and disadvantages to computerized documentation.

Advantages Include

- Enhances the systematic approach to client care through standardized protocols, teaching documents, management and communication.
- Computers are cost-effective and increase the quality of documentation.
- Saves documentation time. Data entry needs to be done only once; the system avoids duplication of entries.
- Increases legibility and accuracy. The program prompts the nurse for information, making the charting more complete, thorough, concise, and organized.
- Provides clear, decisive, and concise key works. Standardized nursing terminology provides usage of consistent key words. Nurses may select choices on a screen that automatically builds a comprehensive record of an event.

- Facilitates statistical analysis of data.
- Enhances critical thinking and decision making by providing access to other data, such as laboratory results that can be correlated with the nurses' assessment data.
- Supports multidisciplinary networking. Information is quickly coordinated and integrated by other departments and all departments have access to data.

Disadvantages Include

- Computer and software may limit the number of terminals at nursing stations.
- Cost of installation.
- Processing speed may be slower at peak usage times.
- Sudden unexpected failure of the computer or software and downtime for routine servicing.

Kardex

A Kardex is a condensed reference tool which includes basic client care information. The Kardex is often used during change-of-shift reports, providing cues regarding pertinent information to discuss or relay. The Kardex may also be utilized as a quick reference throughout the shift.

When a client is admitted onto the nursing unit, data from the physician's admitting orders are generally penciled onto the card. As new physician orders are received, the Kardex is updated to reflect the change. A sample Kardex is shown in Appendix B.

Information contained on the Kardex may vary in different facilities; however, the Kardex often includes data such as:

- Client data: name, age, sex, height, weight
- Emergency data: name of contact person, relationship, address, telephone number
- Daily diagnostic examinations, scheduled examinations or surgery
- Medical diagnoses: admitting and history
- Nursing diagnoses: by priority
- Medical orders: diet, DNR (do not resuscitate) status, isolation, restraints, invasive procedures, vital sign parameters, activity, treatments, such as sitz bath or antiembolytic stockings
- Special therapies: respiratory therapy, physical therapy, occupational therapy
- Routine medications including dosage amounts, times, intravenous solutions and medication, and as-needed medications

REPORTING

Reporting includes verbal communication of facts regarding the client's health status and ongoing care provided. When a report is given, the nurse summarizes the current critical information to facilitate continuity of care. Thought should be given to what data are necessary to report. Table 5:2 identifies an acronym, RECEIVE, with examples of data to include while reporting. Verbal reports may be required in a variety of situations, such as reporting to:

- Oncoming shift personnel with summary reports or walking rounds.
- A receiving unit or facility via telephone when the client is transferred or discharged.
- A superior who is in charge or the health care provider.

TABLE 5:2 Information to Include in a Verbal Report

Reporting: facts, not opinions. Report objectively, accurately, be concise and complete.

Essential information about the client, such as name, age, sex, admission medical diagnosis, and pertinent history data.

Condition: current condition, such as diet, nothing by mouth (NPO), do not resuscitate (DNR) status, response to administered medication, Foley catheter, IV solution and site, orientation, prescribed activity level, fluid restriction, assistance needed by client, current teaching and client response, etc.

Extra medications, such as last prn (as needed) pain medication administered, preoperative medications on call or administered, medications to be given dependent on laboratory values. For example, "Give 20 mEq KCl for potassium <3.0."

Identify priorities relating to care, upcoming procedures, recurring laboratory tests, diagnostic tests completed, and results if known. Identify activities completed and those to be completed.

Values: such as last blood glucose level, vital sign parameters, abnormal vital signs, intake and output amounts, etc.

Exceptional report given!

Nursing Tip

*Always maintain client **confidentiality.** What does this term mean to you?*

CONFIDENTIALITY

Information obtained from or about the client is considered to be *privileged* and, in most cases, cannot be disclosed to a third party. Clients have a legal and ethical right to privacy. As a student or practicing nurse, you have a legal and ethical responsibility for protecting client confidentiality. State laws ensure no one will reveal the client's confidential information without permission. Nurses should not disclose information about the client's status to other clients or staff not involved in the client's care. Nurses should not discuss any client's condition in inappropriate settings, such as the cafeteria or elevator. Nurses must obtain the client's permission before disclosing any information regarding the client, going through the client's personal belongings, performing procedures, and photographing the client.

KEY CONCEPTS

- Implementation is the fourth step in the nursing process. During implementation, nursing interventions are executed and the client's response is observed, communicated, and documented.
- As nurses interact with the client, assessment continues throughout each phase of the nursing process. New data are collected as the client responds to treatment, therapies, and nursing interventions.

- Client responses are reported to other health care professionals involved in the client's care and recorded in the 24-hour client care record (nurse's notes).
- Nurses are ethically and legally obligated to protect client confidentiality and privacy.

STUDENT PRACTICE: DOCUMENTATION
Instructions

Read the brief vignette below.

A. Rewrite data in *narrative* documentation format.
B. Rewrite data in *focus* documentation format.

Complete sentences are not necessary.

Vignette: This morning when day shift began, Mr. James was lying in bed with his eyes closed. When the nurse touched his arm, his skin was warm and dry. Mr. James's respirations were even and unlabored. He did not appear to be in any distress. Report was completed at 0715. When breakfast was served, around 0815, he was watching television. Mr. James complained of muscle spasms to his right lower calf (client recently fractured right tibia). Capillary refill to his right great toe is less than two seconds. Feet are warm to touch and he moves them without difficulty. Skin condition around the cast edges is intact and without evidence of skin breakdown. Dr. Martin was called on the telephone at 0830 to advise of muscle spasms and to request new orders. Dr. Martin was in to see the client at 0955. He wrote an order for Mr. James to receive a new medication to reduce muscle spasms. Discharge orders were written. Mr. James states his wife will arrive within the hour for completion of discharge.

A: Narrative Documentation:

Date	Time	

B: Focus Documentation:

Date	Time	Focus	

STUDENT PRACTICE: CHANGE-OF-SHIFT REPORT
Instructions

Locate Student Practice case scenario for client Mr. C. Gonzales in Chapter 3. Using the data provided, determine information that would be necessary to report during change of shift.

_____

_____

_____

_____

_____

_____

_____

_____

_____

_____

_____

_____

_____

_____

Evaluation

"Evaluation involves analysis of all aspects of phenomena and comparison to a set of standards, criteria, interventions, or expectations to determine effectiveness of the standard, behavior, or intervention. Decisions and changes are made and implemented dependent on evaluation findings."
Lisa O'Steen RN, MSN (Columbus Technical College, ADN Program, Columbus, Georgia)

STANDARD 6: *EVALUATION*

The registered nurse evaluates progress toward attainment of outcomes.

Measurement Criteria

The registered nurse:

- Conducts a systematic, ongoing, and criterion-based evaluation of the outcomes in relation to the structures and processes prescribed by the plan and the indicated timeline.
- Includes the patient and others involved in the care or situation in the evaluative process.
- Evaluates the effectiveness of the planned strategies in relation to patient responses and the attainment of the expected outcomes.
- Documents the results of the evaluation.
- Uses ongoing assessment data to revise the diagnoses, outcomes, the plan, and the implementation as needed.
- Disseminates the results to the patient and others involved in the care or situation, as appropriate, in accordance with state and federal laws and regulations.

(From American Nurses Association. [2004]. *Nursing: Scope and standards of practice. Washington, DC: Author.*)

OBJECTIVES

Upon completion of this chapter, the student should be able to:

- Discuss the purpose of evaluation related to the nursing process.
- Identify characteristics of the evaluation phase and how to document evaluation.
- Discuss the relationship between assessment and evaluation.
- Identify how to evaluate effective goal achievement.
- Discuss when it is necessary to modify, revise, or discontinue portions of the care plan.

KEY TERMS

discontinue	evaluative statement	modification
evaluation	goal attainment	revision

EVALUATION: STEP 5 OF THE NURSING PROCESS

Evaluation is the fifth phase of the nursing process. This step takes a critical look at the *results* of implemented nursing interventions. Although evaluation is the final step described in the nursing process, it is interwoven throughout all other steps. Evaluation involves critical analysis of the plan, beginning with initial data collection and continuing through implementation (Figure 6:1). Like assessment, evaluation is continuous and ongoing. Interventions and client responses are evaluated with questions. For example: Is the client progressing toward goal resolution? Have goals been met? Is this portion of the plan complete and no longer a problem for the client? Have goals been partially met or not met? When the client is not progressing as expected, answers are sought to determine why.

This chapter describes the purpose, characteristics, components, and methods for evaluation. The chapter also discusses evaluation of goal achievement, as well as determination of how and when to revise, modify, or discontinue the care plan.

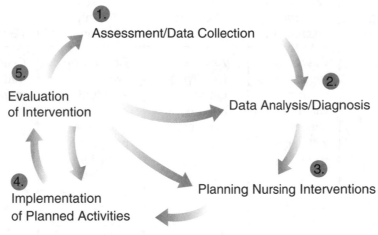

FIGURE 6:1 Relationship of Evaluation to Nursing Process.

Evaluation Purpose

The purpose of the evaluation phase is to estimate the effectiveness of nursing care and the quality of care provided. Nurses evaluate client responses to determine if the care plan is working or how well the care plan is working, and whether the client is progressing toward expected outcomes and goal achievement.

Characteristics of Evaluation

The evaluation phase and the assessment phase are similar in that they are both ongoing. When the client enters the health care continuum, initial assessment data are collected to establish a baseline. Assessment, reassessment, and evaluation continue as *long as care is provided*. Client response is compared to behaviors stated in the goal or expected outcomes, for example, reversal of symptoms, improved energy level, proper use of equipment, or reduced pain. Evaluation focuses on the relationship between the care provided and the client's progress toward goal attainment.

Evaluation is not an end to the nursing process, but a mechanism that assures quality interventions. This phase helps determine if the documented plan is working and if more might be accomplished. The nurse judges the success of the previous steps of the nursing process and examines the client's response to interventions and medical treatment or therapies. Evaluation aids in analysis of the quality of nursing care provided at an institution or agency and helps determine if referral to other resources, consultation, or collaboration may be necessary. The nurse must be sensitive to subtle or obvious changes in the client's physiological condition, emotional status, and behavior. Positive and negative factors are identified which affect the client's response. Inquiries helpful in evaluating the application of the nursing process include:

- Was assessment thorough and accurate?
- Were nursing diagnoses relevant?

> **Nursing Tip**
>
> *Degrees of goal attainment include: the goal is met, partially met, or not met.*

Nursing Diagnosis	Goal Statement	Nursing Interventions	Scientific Rationale	Evaluation
Parenting, altered Related to (R/T) lack of knowledge about child development As evidenced by (AEB): statements of inability to meet child's needs, role inadequacy, frustration	Client will report comfort with role expectations within one week.	Assist with identifying deficits/ alterations in parenting skills.	Counseling involves a mutual exchange of ideas and provides a basis for problem solving.	Client reports that he is more comfortable in role expectations.

FIGURE 6:2 Documenting Evaluation of the Care Plan.

- Did the client and family participate in priority problem identification and goal setting?
- Were goals specific, measurable, and realistic?
- Were expected outcomes achieved?
- Did nursing interventions and actions appropriately address the client's problems?
- Is the plan of care appropriate and accurate?
- Should any portion of the plan be modified or terminated?

Data from the above inquiry are analyzed to determine whether behaviors indicate progress toward goal achievement.

When documented, evaluation is stated in present or past tense. Refer to Figure 6:2 for an example of how evaluation is documented in a care plan.

Review of Goals and Expected Outcomes

A **goal** is the overall desired change in the client's health status or behavior. Goals are phrased in general terms. **Expected outcomes** are stated in more specific terms. Both are directed toward the same destination. Expected outcomes may be thought of as more manageable targets advancing the client toward goal attainment. Goals and expected outcomes express behaviors to be accomplished within a specified time frame. Once the behavior is demonstrated, advancement toward problem resolution is indicated. As hospital stays become shorter, many clients are discharged before all goals are met.

Care Plan Modification

As the client responds to treatment, therapies, and nursing interventions, a change in the care plan may be warranted. Critical thought questions are asked:

- Has the expected outcome occurred?
- Is the client progressing as expected?
- Has there been a change in the client's condition?
- Is the client's health status improving?

Progress toward goal attainment most likely indicates that appropriate interventions were planned and instituted. In this case, the plan of care continues as recorded and the client will continue to be monitored. **Revisions** (rewriting or amending) or **modifications** to the care plan are expected, however, as the client progresses to a higher level of wellness. The care plan is revised or updated to reflect the client's changing needs.

Lack of progress toward goal attainment may indicate the care plan needs modification as well. Unmet and partially met goals reactivate the nursing process sequence as previously discussed. **Modifications** to the care plan are made where needed.

Finally, when goals or desired outcomes are determined as *having been achieved* and the client no longer requires nursing assistance in this area, the nurse **discontinues** that portion of the care plan. Nurses continue to reassess the client for possible return of symptoms. For example, if the nursing diagnosis *Constipation* were resolved and no longer a valid concern to the client, the nurse would continue to assess function of the gastrointestinal tract.

Care Plan Evaluation and Discharge Summary

Length of stay in acute care settings continues to decrease. Preparation for discharge begins at the time of admission. The client's condition and expected outcomes dictate the type of planning required. Some agencies employ personnel with the primary responsibility of teaching or discharge planning for the client. The nurse who is caring for the individual client is responsible for ensuring that all appropriate interventions have been implemented before discharge. Additional services or facilities involved in ongoing health care include rehabilitation facilities, home health care, nursing home care, or health care clinics.

Ideally, when preparing the client for discharge, it is appropriate to evaluate the status of each nursing diagnosis prior to discharge. An **evaluative statement** is written, identifying the client's partial progress toward goal achievement and problem resolution. The care plan is revised for home and follow-up care. This plan is summarized in discharge instructions and documented. Additional assessment and documentation criteria may be required according to the policy and procedures of individual facilities.

KEY CONCEPTS

- Evaluation is the fifth step of the nursing process. Although it is the final step, evaluation is interwoven throughout the entire nursing process sequence. Evaluation is continuous and cyclic in nature.
- The purpose of evaluation is to judge the effectiveness of chosen interventions, nursing care, and the quality of care provided.
- As evaluation takes place, assessment of the client continues. Evaluation of goal attainment compares the client's behavior or response to the behavior or response specified in the stated goal. It is this behavior and stated time frame that make goals measurable.

- Degrees of goal attainment include: the goal was met, partially met, or not met.
- As the client progresses toward a higher level of wellness, revisions or modifications to the care plan are expected. When specific problems have been resolved and no longer require intervention from the nurse, this portion of the care plan may be discontinued. Evaluation in the previously problematic area continues for possible return of signs or symptoms.

STUDENT PRACTICE: EVALUATION

Instructions

Answer the following questions:

1. What three essential cognitive skills are practiced in all steps of the nursing process? Define each skill.

   A. _____

   _____

   _____

   B. _____

   _____

   _____

   _____

   C. _____

   _____

   _____

   _____

2. Give one example of how the nurse may employ critical thinking in the following vignette: As the nurse entered the client's room, the client was holding her midchest or sternum area. The client was breathing faster than usual.

   _____

   _____

   _____

   _____

   _____

   _____

   _____

   _____

3. What is the difference between assessment and evaluation?

_____

_____

_____

_____

_____

_____

_____

4. What are the similarities between assessment and evaluation?

_____

_____

_____

_____

_____

_____

_____

5. How is evaluation documented on the care plan?

_____

_____

_____

_____

_____

_____

6. What is the purpose of evaluation?

_____

_____

_____

_____

_____

_____

_____

7. What does goal attainment mean in relation to evaluation and the nursing process?

_____

_____

_____

_____

_____

_____

_____

_____

8. When is the care plan or portions of the care plan revised, modified, or discontinued?

_____

_____

_____

_____

_____

_____

_____

_____

_____

_____

_____

Putting It All Together!

"In watching diseases, both in private houses and in public hospitals, the thing that strikes the experienced observer most forcibly is this, that the symptoms of the sufferings generally considered to be inevitable and incident to the disease are very often not symptoms of the disease at all, but of something quite different – of the want of fresh air, or of light, or of warmth, or of quiet, or of cleanliness, or of punctuality and care in the administration of diet, of each or of all of these."

Florence Nightingale

OBJECTIVES

Upon completion of this chapter, the student should be able to:

- Apply the steps of the nursing process to the provided scenario.
- Discuss each step of the nursing process, actions taken by nurses during each step, and the rationale of each action as it is applied.
- Identify how critical thinking is an important element of the nursing process.

APPLICATION OF THE NURSING PROCESS

The nursing process is a cyclic, ongoing method of providing client-centered care. It is a tool used by nurses to promote organization and utilization of the steps to achieve desired outcomes, that is, goal attainment and problem resolution.

As the client enters the health care system, nurses are involved in decision making. Care is planned for the client based on data continuously collected and analyzed. Initial data collected become the database used for comparison of future data.

Nurses use skills vital to all steps of the nursing process: critical thinking, problem solving, and decision making. Critical thinking is a purposeful thought process, in which deliberate questions are asked in search of meaning of data. Nurses solve problems by analyzing collected data in order to understand and make decisions regarding client needs. Decisions are made based on the nurse's understanding of scientifically based theories and knowledge of standards. These skills and others are employed as nurses interact with clients. Each interaction is an opportunity for the nurse to assess and evaluate client responses to care and medical treatment, as well as the effectiveness of care.

This chapter presents a review discussion of the nursing process. The nursing process steps are applied to a sample scenario, as if providing care to a client. A final care plan appears at the end of the chapter (Figure 7:1).

STEP 1: ASSESSMENT

Assessment includes collection, validation, organization, and interpretation of data. Initial data gathered during an interview, physical assessment, and review of diagnostic studies become the client database. This data may be used for comparison as additional data are collected. Once the client enters the health care system, other sources of data may include nursing records, medical records, verbal and written consultations, relevant literature regarding the client's illness, standards indicating normal functioning against which the client is compared, and other members of the health care team working with the client. Assessment is a continuous process of collecting data to identify needs of the client and perpetuates as long as there is a need for health care.

Two categories of data are collected, subjective and objective. *Subjective* data include statements made by the client, such as feelings, perceptions, or concerns. *Objective* data include signs which are observable, measurable, or felt by someone other than the person experiencing them. Each category complements and clarifies the other.

Collected assessment data are recorded using various tools designed for that purpose. Tools should consider all aspects of the client including physical, emotional, social, spiritual, and economic well-being.

As data are collected, verified, and validated for accuracy, the nurse assigns meaning and groups data into clusters. Data clustering is used to determine the relatedness of facts, to find patterns, and to determine if further data are needed. Related subjective and objective data are clustered together supporting the fact that a health problem exists that requires intervention.

Client Scenario

General Information

Name: Mrs. L. N.
Age: 78 years   **Gender:** Female   **Race/Ethnicity:** African American
Admitting Medical Diagnosis: Bronchitis
Admitting Weight/Height/Vital Signs: Weight 122 pounds; height 60 inches; blood pressure 148/74; pulse 116 beats per minute; temperature 102.2°F; respiratory rate 26 breaths per minute
Perception of Reason for Admission: Chest discomfort, dyspnea, cough, fatigue, fever
Allergies: No known food or drug allergies
Current Medications: No prescription medications; takes acetaminophen for headaches

Assessment Data

Neuro/Orientation: Answers all questions appropriately; alert, oriented to person, time, place. No sensory deficits.

Oxygenation: Reports progressive difficulty breathing over last two days; oxygen is being administered via nasal cannula at two liters per minute; states she is a non-smoker, however her husband has smoked cigarettes for over 20 years; breath sounds with crackles in bilateral lower lobes; inspiratory and expiratory wheezing to bilateral mid and lower lungs; ineffective, nonproductive cough; increased use of accessory muscles; apical pulse 116 beats per minute, regular; peripheral pulses equal, regular, strong bilaterally; skin color with pale pink-yellow undertones; capillary refill sluggish, greater than two seconds; oxygen saturation is low; reports chest discomfort which increases with deep inhalation and cough. Mrs. N. is restless and has difficulty vocalizing.

Temperature: 102.2°F; reports elevated temperature and chills for previous three days.

Nutritional/Fluid: Denies difficulty chewing or swallowing food, normal appetite; has maintained oral fluid intake; no nausea or vomiting; skin is elastic with instant recoil.

Elimination: Voids without difficulty five to seven times daily; reports normal bowel pattern.

Rest/Sleep: usually retires around 9:00 p.m. and sleeps until 5:00 a.m., however, is experiencing increased fatigue; does not feel rested after full nights sleep; no energy.

Pain Avoidance: Reports chest discomfort when she coughs or inhales deeply. Unable to rate discomfort or describe; mild headache; muscle aches.

Activity: States she usually bowls twice weekly with her husband and previously able to perform all activities of daily living (ADLs) without difficulty, however, since becoming ill, experiences exhaustion and becomes short of breath with physical exertion. Observed dyspnea with exertion while transferring from wheelchair to bed.

Additional Data: Denies visual or hearing problems; pupils equal and reactive to light; skin is intact. Saline lock is in her right hand and sight is without erythema or edema.

Laboratory/Diagnostic Reports: Chest radiograph reveals an acute infiltrate in left lower lung field; routine laboratory tests include CBC, serum electrolytes, renal function and arterial blood gases have been drawn with results pending.

This scenario represents initial assessment data collected from the client's interview and physical assessment. The nurse utilizes a data collection format approved for his or her facility. As the nurse collects data, questions are asked to verify or validate data when necessary. The nurse is now ready to organize the data, first by separating abnormal objective data (measurements and observations) from subjective data (statements and feelings that only the client can identify). Finally, the nurse clusters data to determine their relatedness and confirm that health problems or risk problems exist.

Subjective and Objective Data

Subjective Data

- Progressive difficulty breathing
- Report of elevated temperature and chills
- Chest discomfort with cough or inhalation
- Headache, muscle aches
- Fatigue
- Husband smokes (environmental exposure)
- No energy, not rested
- Dyspnea with exertion

Objective Data

- Blood pressure 148/74
- Pulse 116 per minute
- Temperature 102.2°F
- Respiratory rate 26 per minute with use of accessory muscles
- Oxygen via nasal cannula
- Crackles to bilateral lower lobes; wheezing in bilateral lobes
- Consolidation in left lower lobe with radiograph revealing infiltrate
- Ineffective nonproductive cough
- Capillary refill sluggish
- Oxygen saturation low on room air
- Restless
- Difficulty vocalizing
- Observed dyspnea with exertion

Clustering Data

Activity	Respiratory	Physical Regulation
<ul><li>Fatigue, does not feel rested after sleeping</li><li>Muscle aches</li><li>Chest discomfort with cough and inhalation</li><li>Dyspnea with exertion</li><li>Restlessness</li></ul>	<ul><li>Difficulty in breathing</li><li>Ineffective nonproductive cough</li><li>Respiratory rate increased, use of accessory muscles to breathe</li><li>Oxygen saturation low on room air, need of supplemental oxygen</li><li>Radiograph revealing infiltrate, consolidation in left lower lung, crackles auscultated in bilateral lower lobes; wheezing in bilateral lobes</li><li>Second-hand smoke exposure</li><li>Difficulty vocalizing</li><li>Restlessness</li></ul>	<ul><li>Elevated temperature, chills</li><li>Pulse 116 per minute</li><li>Elevated blood pressure</li><li>Dyspnea with exertion</li><li>Increased respiratory rate</li><li>Headache</li></ul>

As you can see, objective and subjective data compliment and clarify each other. Once data are clustered, it becomes evident that health problems and risk problems exist. The care plan will be developed from initial and ongoing data collection.

STEP 2: DIAGNOSIS

Diagnosis involves critical thought and judgment to analyze, organize, and interpret assessment data. Problems, risk problems, and strengths are identified and labeled with NANDA nursing diagnoses. Once labeled, the nursing diagnosis communicates specific health care needs about the client to other members of the health care team involved in care.

The data collection tool used in the scenario provides information pertaining to specific areas of functioning: comfort, respiratory function, and regulatory function. Review the list of clustered data under each category where actual problems are discovered during the assessment step. Information should be analyzed, interpreted, and labeled with nursing diagnoses.

The following is a list of actual or risk nursing diagnoses, related to (R/T) risk factors, and defining characteristics, which will be included in the care plan. Locate each nursing diagnosis in Appendix A and read the definition. Does the definition apply to Mrs. N.?

- *Gas Exchange, Impaired*
  R/T: ventilation perfusion imbalance
  As evidenced by (AEB): tachycardia, hypoxia, dyspnea, abnormal rate and depth of breathing
- *Activity Intolerance* (Level III)
  R/T: imbalance between oxygen supply and demand
  AEB: report of increasing fatigue and exhaustion, dyspnea with exertion, increased heart rate, respiratory rate, and blood pressure

Impaired Gas Exchange and *Activity Intolerance* are priority nursing diagnoses labeling *actual* client health problems. She is exhibiting signs and symptoms in response to her medical condition. The client may be *at risk* for additional problems if her condition worsens.

STEP 3: PLANNING AND OUTCOME IDENTIFICATION

Planning the care for the client involves several steps:

- Identifying priority problems
- Setting realistic goals and expected outcomes
- Determining nursing interventions and scientific rationale
- Communicating and documenting the care plan

The planning step should involve discussing the plan with the client for input and collaboration. This encourages client participation and promotes the client's sense of control. Careful, effective planning advocates and ensures delivery of quality care.

Determining priorities involves analyzing data to discover situations requiring immediate attention. The client often communicates this during the interview or assessment. Consider Maslow's hierarchy of needs. The basic physiological needs include oxygenation, nutrition, hydration, elimination, body temperature maintenance, and pain avoidance.

In our scenario, Mrs. N. demonstrated outstanding signs and symptoms in areas of pain avoidance, oxygenation, and activity. After collaboration, she confirmed her respiratory status as the priority problem, at the moment.

Establishing goals and expected outcomes follow priority problem identification. One overall goal is determined for each nursing diagnosis. Goals are guidelines which help to individualize nursing interventions. Goals give direction to the care plan and focus on the etiology of the problem. *Goals* are general statements indicating the intent or desired change in the client's health status, function, or behavior. *Expected outcomes* are stated in specific terms, describing methods through which the goal will be achieved.

Required components of goals include the subject (client), behavior, criteria of performance, and time frame. An optional component is the condition, referring to the aid which facilitates the performance. Goals and expected outcomes must be realistic. Review the following goals/expected outcomes for Mrs. N. *Can you identify each component of the goal statement?*

Nursing diagnosis: Gas Exchange, Impaired. R/T: ventilation perfusion imbalance. AEB: tachycardia, hypoxia, dyspnea, abnormal rate and depth of breathing.

Goal/client outcomes: Mrs. N. will demonstrate improved ventilation and absence of symptoms of respiratory distress within 24 hours.

Nursing diagnosis: Activity Intolerance (Level III). R/T: imbalance between oxygen supply and demand. AEB: report of increasing fatigue and exhaustion, dyspnea with exertion, increased heart rate, respiratory rate, and blood pressure.

Goal/client outcomes: Mrs. N. will report improved ability to perform activities without experiencing dyspnea within 48 hours after initiation of medical/nursing treatment.

Planning Nursing Interventions

Nursing interventions are activities planned and executed by the nursing team which benefit the client in a predictable manner. Interventions are selected based on scientific principles and knowledge of behavioral and physical sciences. Nurses use deliberate thought, decision making, and problem solving to determine actions which will aid in elimination, prevention, or reduction of the cause of the problem or nursing diagnosis. Nursing interventions are developed from the etiology of each nursing diagnosis. Generally, several interventions should be identified for each goal.

Interventions are selected based on the nurse's understanding of scientific principle and psychosocial or developmental theories. Understanding of the human body and mind allows for certain expected responses when interventions are carried out. The term *scientific rationale* is the underlying reason for choosing a specific intervention. *Do you remember?*

Explain the process of locating scientific rationales.

_____

_____

_____

Can you list four or more sources?

_____

_____

Describe steps taken when locating scientific rationale.

_____

_____

_____

Nursing interventions and scientific rationale for our scenario follow:

Nursing diagnosis: Gas Exchange, Impaired. R/T: ventilation perfusion imbalance. AEB: tachycardia, hypoxia, dyspnea, abnormal rate and depth of breathing.

Goal/client outcomes: Mrs. N. will demonstrate improved ventilation and absence of symptoms of respiratory distress within 24 hours.

Nursing interventions and *scientific rationales:*

1. Maintain elevated head of bed. *Promotes optimal chest expansion and drainage of secretions.*
2. Encourage and maintain adequate fluid intake. *Helps to mobilize lung secretions and improve expectoration.*
3. Administer prescribed medications, such as antibiotics. *To treat underlying condition and improve respiratory status.*
4. Encourage adequate rest and promote calm environment. *Helps limit oxygen needs/consumption.*

Nursing diagnosis: Activity Intolerance (Level III). R/T: imbalance between oxygen supply and demand. AEB: report of increasing fatigue and exhaustion, dyspnea with exertion, increased heart rate, respiratory rate, and blood pressure.

Goal/client outcomes: Mrs. N. will report improved ability to perform activities without experiencing dyspnea within 48 hours after initiation of medical/nursing treatment.

Nursing interventions and *scientific rationales:*

1. Evaluate current limitations as compared to usual activity status. *Provides a comparative baseline.*
2. Provide adequate rest periods between activities. *To limit fatigue and to prevent overexertion.*
3. Assist with activities and encourage patient to increase activity levels gradually. *Conserves and improves energy level.*

Once the plan of care is developed it is shared with other members of the health care team involved in caring for the client. The plan is communicated verbally and through written documentation. The care plan records health care needs, coordinates nursing care, promotes continuity of care, encourages communication within the health care team, and promotes quality nursing care.

STEP 4: IMPLEMENTATION

During *implementation,* planned nursing interventions are executed. This step begins with assessment and evaluation of the client prior to initiating care. Each interaction with the client is an opportunity to assess, collect ongoing data, and compare data to the client's baseline. Nurses apply scientific knowledge and understanding, analytical skills, and deliberate thought to interpret ongoing data collection. Priority interventions are carried out first. However, nurses may perform interventions for more than one problem at the same time.

The nurse is legally required to record all interventions implemented as well as observations related to the client's response to treatments. Written documentation provides a legal record and can be reviewed by other health care team members involved in the patient's care.

STEP 5: EVALUATION

The *evaluation* phase measures the effectiveness of nursing care and the quality of care provided. However, evaluation, like assessment, is not a static activity, but ongoing and cyclic, never ceasing. As interventions are carried out, client *responses* are evaluated and the client is reassessed. Questions are asked about the appropriateness and effectiveness of the intervention and the client's response to medical treatment, therapies, and nursing interventions. Are goals being met? If not, answers are sought to determine why.

Evaluation of the care plan focuses on changes in the client's health status, that is, if the client is progressing toward goal attainment. As the client's health status changes, the care plan is revised to reflect the changing needs.

Lack of progress toward goal attainment may indicate the care plan needs revisions or modifications. The nursing process sequence is reactivated and assessment begins again. Once again, collected data are analyzed, organized, and interpreted. All planning is compared to that previously determined, searching for omissions or inaccuracies. A revised care plan is developed and executed.

During evaluation, when goals and expected outcomes are determined as having been achieved and the client no longer requires nursing assistance in this area, this portion of the care plan is discontinued. Nurses will continue to assess and evaluate the client for possible return of symptoms.

The completed care plan for Mrs. N is provided in Figure 7:1.

STUDENT PRACTICE

Instructions

Read the case scenario and apply the five steps of the nursing process. Identify three appropriate nursing diagnoses (with *R/T* and *AEB* or *risk factors*). For each nursing diagnosis provide one goal/expected outcome, three nursing interventions with scientific rationale, and one evaluative statement. The care plan form is attached.

General Information

Name: Mr. Stephen (Tipper) Carlson
Age: 45 years   **Gender:** Male   **Race/Ethnicity:** Caucasian
Admitting Medical Diagnosis: S/P Motor vehicle accident (MVA) with fractured pelvis and multiple contusions
Admitting Weight/Height/Vital Signs: Weight 165 pounds; height 67 inches; temperature 99.0°F; blood pressure 144/88; heart rate 90 beats per minute; respiratory rate 22 breaths per minute.
Client's Perception of Reason for Admission: "I was in a car accident."
Allergies: None
Current Medications: No prescription medications; no over-the-counter (OTC) medications.
Past Medical History: Appendectomy at age eight years.

Nursing Diagnosis	Goal/Expected Outcomes	Nursing Interventions	Scientific Rationale	Evaluation
Gas Exchange, Impaired R/T: ventilation perfusion imbalance AEB: tachycardia, hypoxia, dyspnea, abnormal rate and depth of breathing	Mrs. N. will demonstrate improved ventilation and absence of symptoms of respiratory distress within 24 hours.	1. Maintain elevated head of bed at all times. 2. Encourage and maintain adequate fluid intake. 3. Administer prescribed medications, such as antibiotics. 4. Encourage adequate rest and promote calm environment.	1. Promotes optimal chest expansion and drainage of secretions. 2. Helps to mobilize lung secretions and improve expectoration of secretions. 3. To treat underlying condition and improve respiratory status. 4. Helps limit oxygen needs/consumption.	Pulse oximeter reading 98% oxygen saturation throughout shift. Respiratory rate 20 breaths per minute. Mrs. N. denies shortness of breath.
Activity Intolerance (Level III) R/T: imbalance between oxygen supply and demand AEB: report of increasing fatigue and exhaustion, dyspnea with exertion, increased heart rate, respiratory rate, and blood pressure	Mrs. N. will report improved ability to perform activities without experiencing dyspnea within 48 hours after initiation of medical/nursing treatment.	1. Evaluate current limitations as compared to usual activity status. 2. Provide adequate rest periods between activities. 3. Assist with activities and encourage patient to increase activity levels gradually.	1. Provides a comparative baseline. 2. To limit fatigue and to prevent overexertion. 3. Conserves and improves energy level.	Mrs. N. is able to assist in self care without becoming short of breath.

Note: each required component is included in this goal statement

Note: evaluation is reported in present or past tense.

Note: each nursing intervention requires scientific rationale

FIGURE 7:1 Documented Care Plan for Mrs. N.

Assessment Data

Neuro/Orientation: Alert, oriented to person, time, place.

Cardiovascular: Denies dyspnea; states he is a nonsmoker; breath sounds clear to auscultation bilaterally; no cough; apical pulse 90 beats per minute and regular; peripheral pulses equal, regular and strong bilaterally; skin warm, pink, and dry; capillary refill less than two seconds.

Nutritional/Fluid: Denies difficulty chewing or swallowing food; normal appetite; no nausea or vomiting; skin is elastic with instant recoil; prescribed nothing by mouth (NPO) at this time.

Elimination: Foley catheter to gravity drainage with clear, light yellow urine; reports usually bowel elimination pattern as once each day, however, has had no bowel movement for four days; abdominal bowel sounds are hypoactive in all four quadrants.

Rest/Sleep: Usually retires around 10:00 p.m. and sleeps until 5:00 a.m.

Pain Avoidance: Reports severe pain to pelvic area, rated as "7" on a scale of zero to ten, described as "intense, ripping sensation with muscle spasms;" muscle aches throughout body.

Activity: Previously active, no deficits. At this time, physician prescribed complete bed rest with continuous pelvic traction.

Additional Data: No visual or hearing deficits; pupils equal and reactive to light; superficial wounds noted to left, lateral forearm, wrist, and hand, with no erythema, no edema. Ecchymosis (bruising) observed to left, lateral pelvic and abdominal regions. Abdomen is soft with mild tenderness to left upper and lower abdomen when lightly palpated.

Laboratory/Diagnostic Reports: Computed tomography (CT) reveals fractured left pelvis. Laboratory findings are unremarkable.

Appendix A

2005–2006 NORTH AMERICAN NURSING DIAGNOSIS ASSOCIATION (NANDA)

Diagnoses, Definitions, Risk Factors or Related Factors, and Defining Characteristics

Reprinted with permission of North American Nursing Diagnosis Association, 2005, Philadelphia: NANDA.

Activity intolerance

Definition: individual has insufficient physiological or psychological energy to endure or complete required or desired daily activities

Related factors: bedrest or immobility; generalized weakness; imbalance between oxygen supply/demand; sedentary lifestyle

Defining characteristics: verbal report of fatigue or weakness; abnormal heart rate or blood pressure response to activity; electrocardiographic changes reflecting arrhythmias or ischemia; exertional discomfort or dyspnea

Activity intolerance, risk for

Definition: at risk for experiencing insufficient physiological or psychological energy to endure or complete required or desired daily activities

Risk factors: inexperience with the activity; presence of circulatory/respiratory problems; history of previous intolerance; deconditioned status

Adaptive capacity, intracranial, decreased

Definition: intracranial fluid dynamic mechanisms that normally compensate for increases in intracranial volumes are compromised, resulting in repeated, disproportionate increases in intracranial pressure in response to a variety of noxious and non-noxious stimuli

Related factors: decreased cerebral perfusion pressure ≤50–60 mm Hg; sustained increase in ICP ≥ 10–15 mm Hg; systemic hypotension with intracranial hypertension; brain injuries

Defining characteristics: repeated increases of greater than 10 mm Hg for more than five minutes following any of a variety of external stimuli; baseline ICP ≥ 10 mm Hg; disproportionate increase in ICP following single environmental or nursing maneuver stimulus; elevated P_2 ICP waveform; volume pressure response test variation (volume-pressure ratio >2, pressure-volume index <10); wide amplitude ICP waveform

Adjustment, impaired
Definition: inability to modify life style/behavior in a manner consistent with a change in health status
Related factors: low state of optimism; intense emotional state; negative attitudes toward health behavior; absence of intent to change behavior; multiple stressors; absence of social support for changed beliefs and practices; disability or health status change requiring change in life style; lack of motivation to change behaviors
Defining characteristics: denial of health status change; failure to achieve optimal sense of control; failure to take actions that would prevent further health problems; demonstration of nonacceptance of health status change

Airway clearance, ineffective
Definition: inability to clear secretions or obstructions from the respiratory tract to maintain a clear airway
Related factors:
Environmental: smoking; smoke inhalation; second-hand smoke
Obstructed airway: airway spasm; retained secretions; excessive mucus; presence of artificial airway; foreign body in airway; secretions in the bronchi; exudate in the alveoli
Physiological: neuromuscular dysfunction; hyperplasia of the bronchial walls; chronic obstructive pulmonary disease; infection; asthma; allergic airways
Defining characteristics: dyspnea; diminished breath sounds; orthopnea; adventitious breath sounds (rales, crackles, rhonchi, wheezes); ineffective or absent cough; sputum production; cyanosis; difficulty vocalizing; wide-eyed (look); changes in respiratory rate and rhythm; restlessness

Allergy response, latex
Definition: an allergic response to natural latex rubber products
Related factors: no immune mechanism; response
Defining characteristics:
Type I Reactions: immediate reactions (<1 hour) to latex proteins (can be life threatening); contact urticaria progressing to generalized symptoms; edema of the lips, tongue, uvula, and/or throat; shortness of breath, tightness in chest, wheezing, bronchospasm leading to respiratory arrest; hypotension, syncope, cardiac arrest
May also include: orofacial characteristics (edema of sclera or eyelids; erythema and/or itching of the eyes; tearing of the eyes; nasal congestion, itching, and/or erythema; rhinorrhea; facial erythema; facial itching; oral itching); gastrointestinal characteristics (abdominal pain; nausea); generalized characteristics (flushing; general discomfort; generalized edema; increasing complaint of total body warmth; restlessness)
Type II Reactions: delayed onset (hours); eczema; irritation; reaction to additives (e.g., thiurams, carbmates) causes discomfort; redness
Irritant Reactions: erythema; chapped or cracked skin; blisters

Allergy response, risk for latex
Definition: at risk for allergic response to natural latex rubber products
Risk factors: multiple surgical procedures, especially from infancy (e.g., spina bifida); allergies to bananas, avocados, tropical fruits, kiwi, chestnuts; professionals with daily exposure to latex

(e.g., medicine, nursing, dentistry); conditions associated with continuous or intermittent catheterization; history of reactions to latex (e.g., balloons, condoms, gloves); allergies to poinsettia plants; history of allergies and asthma

Anxiety

Definition: vague, uneasy feeling of discomfort or dread accompanied by an autonomic response (the source often nonspecific or unknown to the individual); a feeling of apprehension caused by anticipation of danger. It is an altering signal that warns of impending danger and enables the individual to take measures to deal with threat.

Related factors: exposure to toxins; threat to or change in: role status, health status, interaction patterns, role function, environment, economic status; unconscious conflict about essential values/goals of life; familial association/heredity; unmet needs; interpersonal transmission/contagion; threat of death; threat to self-concept; unconscious conflict about essential values/goals of life; stress; substance abuse

Defining characteristics:

Behavioral: diminished productivity; scanning and vigilance; poor eye contact; restlessness; glancing about; extraneous movement (e.g., foot shuffling, hand/arm movements); expressed concerns due to change in life events; insomnia; fidgeting

Affective: regretful; irritability; anguish; scared; jittery; overexcited; painful and persistent increased helplessness; rattled; uncertainty; increased wariness; focus on self; feelings of inadequacy; fearful; distressed; anxious; worried, apprehensive

Physiological: voice quivering, trembling/hand tremors; shakiness; increased respiration (sympathetic); urinary urgency (parasympathetic); increased pulse (sympathetic); pupil dilation (sympathetic); increased reflexes (sympathetic); abdominal pain (parasympathetic); sleep disturbance (parasympathetic); tingling in extremities (parasympathetic); cardiovascular excitation (sympathetic); increased perspiration; facial tension; anorexia (sympathetic); heart pounding (sympathetic); diarrhea (parasympathetic); fatigue (parasympathetic); dry mouth (sympathetic); decreased pulse (parasympathetic); facial flushing (sympathetic); superficial vasoconstriction (sympathetic); twitching (sympathetic); decreased blood pressure (parasympathetic); nausea (parasympathetic); urinary frequency (parasympathetic); faintness (parasympathetic); respiratory difficulties (sympathetic); increased blood pressure (sympathetic)

Cognitive: blocking of thought; confusion; preoccupation; forgetfulness; rumination; impaired attention; decreased perceptual field; fear of unspecific consequences; tendency to blame others; difficulty concentrating; diminished ability to problem solve; diminished ability to learn; awareness of physiologic symptoms

Anxiety, death

Definition: apprehension, worry, or fear related to death or dying

Related factors: to be developed

Defining characteristics: worrying about the impact of one's own death or significant others; powerless over issues related to dying; fear of loss of physical and/or mental abilities when dying; anticipated pain related to dying; deep sadness; fear of the process of dying; concerns of overworking the caregiver as terminal illness incapacitates self; concern about meeting one's creator or feeling doubtful about the existence of a God or Higher Being; total loss of control over any aspect of one's own death; negative death images or unpleasant thoughts about any event related to death or dying; fear of delayed demise;

fear of premature death because it prevents the accomplishment of important life goals; worrying about being the cause of other's grief and suffering; fear of leaving family alone after death; fear of developing a terminal illness; denial of one's own mortality or impending death

Aspiration, risk for
Definition: at risk for entry of gastrointestinal secretions, oropharyngeal secretions, solids, or fluids into tracheobronchial passages
Risk factors: increased intragastric pressure; tube feedings; situations hindering elevation of upper body; reduced level of consciousness; presence of tracheostomy or endotracheal tube; medication administration; wired jaws; increased gastric residual; incomplete lower esophageal sphincter; impaired swallowing; gastrointestinal tubes; facial, oral, neck surgery or trauma; depressed cough and gag reflexes; decreased gastrointestinal motility; delayed gastric emptying

Attachment, risk for impaired parent/infant/child
Definition: disruption of the interactive process between parent/significant other, child, and infant that fosters the development of a protective and nurturing reciprocal relationship
Risk factors: physical barriers; anxiety associated with the parent role; substance abuse; premature infant, ill infant/child, who is unable to effectively initiate parental contact due to altered behavioral organization; lack of privacy; inability of parents to meet personal needs; separation

Autonomic dysreflexia
Definition: life-threatening, uninhibited sympathetic response of the nervous system to a noxious stimulus after a spinal cord injury at T7 or above
Related factors: bladder distension; bowel distention; lack of patient and caregiver knowledge; skin irritation
Defining characteristics: pallor (below the injury); paroxysmal hypertension (sudden periodic elevated blood pressure with systolic pressure >140 mmHg and diastolic pressure >90 mmHg); red splotches on skin (above the injury); bradycardia or tachycardia (heart rate <60 or >100 beats per minute); diaphoresis (above the injury); headache (a diffuse pain in different portions of the head and not confined to any nerve distribution area); blurred vision; chest pain; chilling conjunctival congestion; Horner's syndrome (contraction of the pupil, partial ptosis of the eyelid, enophthalmos and sometimes loss of sweating over the affected side of the fact); metallic taste in mouth; nasal congestion; paresthesia; pilomotor reflex (goose-flesh formation when skin is cooled)

Autonomic dysreflexia, risk for
Definition: at risk for life-threatening, uninhibited response of the sympathetic nervous system, post spinal shock, in an individual with spinal cord injury or lesion at T6 or above (has been demonstrated in patients with injuries at T7 and T8)
Risk factors: an injury/lesion at T6 or above and at least one of the following noxious stimuli:
Neurological stimuli: painful/irritating stimuli below level of injury
Urological stimuli: bladder distention; detrusor sphincter dyssynergia; bladder spasm; instrumentation or surgery; epididymitis; urethritis; urinary tract injection; calculi; cystitis; catheterization

Gastrointestinal stimuli: bowel distention; fecal impaction; digital stimulation; suppositories; hemorrhoids; difficult passage of feces; constipation; enemas; GI system pathology; gastric ulcers; esophageal reflux; gallstones
Reproductive stimuli: menstruation; sexual intercourse; pregnancy; labor and delivery; ovarian cyst; ejaculation
Musculoskeletal-integumentary stimuli: cutaneous stimulation (e.g., pressure ulcer, ingrown toenail, dressings, burns, rash); pressure over bony prominences or genitalia; heterotrophic bone; spasm; fractures; range-of-motion exercises; wounds; sunburns
Regulatory stimuli: temperature fluctuations; extreme environmental temperatures
Situational stimuli: positioning; constrictive clothing (e.g., straps, stockings, shoes); drug reactions (e.g., decongestants, sympathomimetics, vasoconstrictors, narcotic withdrawal); surgical procedure
Cardiac/pulmonary problems: pulmonary emboli; deep vein thrombosis

Body image disturbed
Definition: confusion in mental picture of one's physical self
Related factors: psychosocial; biophysical; cognitive/perceptual; cultural or spiritual; developmental changes; illness; trauma or injury; surgery; illness treatment
Defining characteristics: nonverbal response to actual or perceived change in structure and/or function; verbalization of feelings that reflect an altered view of one's body in appearance, structure, or function; verbalization of perceptions that reflect an altered view of one's body in appearance, structure, or function; behaviors of avoidance, monitoring, or acknowledgment of one's body
Objective: missing body part; trauma to nonfunctioning part; not touching body part; hiding or overexposing body part (intentional or unintentional); actual change in [body] structure and/or function; change in social involvement; change in ability to estimate spatial relationship of body to environment; extension of body boundary to incorporate environmental objects; not looking at body part
Subjective: refusal to verify actual change; preoccupation with change or loss; personalization of part or loss by name; depersonalization of [body] part or loss by impersonal pronouns; extension of body boundary to incorporate environmental objects; negative feelings about body (e.g., feelings of helplessness, hopelessness, or powerlessness); verbalization of change in lifestyle; focus on past strength, function, or appearance; fear of rejection or of reaction by others; emphasis on remaining strengths and heightened achievement

Body temperature, risk for imbalanced
Definition: at risk for failure to maintain body temperature within normal range.
Risk factors: altered metabolic rate; illness or trauma affecting temperature regulation; medications causing vasoconstriction or vasodilation; inappropriate clothing for environmental temperature; inactivity or vigorous activity; extremes of weight; extremes of ages; dehydration; sedation; exposure to cold/cool or warm/hot environments

Breastfeeding, effective
Definition: mother-infant dyad/family exhibits adequate proficiency and satisfaction with breastfeeding process

Related factors: infant gestational age greater than 34 weeks; supportive source; normal infant oral structure; maternal confidence; basic breastfeeding knowledge; normal breast structure
Defining characteristics: effective mother/infant communication patterns; regular and sustained suckling/swallowing at the breast; appropriate infant weight pattern for age; infant content after feeding; mother able to position infant at breast to promote a successful latch-on response; signs and/or symptoms of oxytocin release; adequate infant elimination patterns for age; eagerness of infant to nurse; maternal verbalization of satisfaction with the breastfeeding process

Breastfeeding, ineffective
Definition: dissatisfaction or difficulty a mother, infant, or child experiences with the breastfeeding process
Related factors: nonsupportive partner/family; previous breast surgery; infant receiving supplemental feedings with artificial nipple; prematurity; previous history of breastfeeding failure; poor infant sucking reflex; maternal breast anomaly; maternal anxiety or ambivalence; interruption in breastfeeding; infant anomaly; knowledge deficit
Defining characteristics: unsatisfactory breastfeeding process; nonsustained suckling at the breast; resisting latching on; unresponsive to other comfort measures; persistence of sore nipples beyond the first week of breastfeeding; observable signs of inadequate infant intake; insufficient emptying of each breast per feeding; infant inability to attach on to maternal breast correctly; infant arching and crying at the breast; infant exhibiting fussiness and crying within the first hour after breastfeeding; actual or perceived inadequate milk supply; no observable signs of oxytocin release; insufficient opportunity for suckling at the breast

Breastfeeding, interrupted
Definition: break in the continuity of the breastfeeding process as a result of inability or inadvisability to put baby to breast for feeding
Related factors: contraindications to breastfeeding; maternal employment; maternal or infant illness; need to abruptly wean infant; prematurity
Defining characteristics: infant does not receive nourishment at the breast for some or all of feedings; lack of knowledge regarding expression and storage of breast milk; maternal desire to maintain lactation and provide (or eventually provide) her breast milk for her infant's nutritional needs; separation of mother and infant

Breathing pattern, ineffective
Definition: inspiration and/or expiration that does not provide adequate ventilation
Related factors: hyperventilation; hypoventilation syndrome; bony deformity; pain; chest wall deformity; anxiety; decreased energy/fatigue; neuromuscular dysfunction; musculoskeletal impairment; perception/cognitive impairment; obesity; spinal cord injury; body position; neurological immaturity; respiratory muscle fatigue
Defining characteristics: decreased inspiratory/expiratory pressure; decreased minute ventilation; use of accessory muscles to breathe; nasal flaring; dyspnea; orthopnea; altered chest excursion; shortness of breath; assumption of three-point position; pursed lip breathing; prolonged expiration phases; increased anterior-posterior diameter; respiratory rate/min (infants: age 0–12 mo <25 or >60; children: 1–4 yr <20

or >30; children: 5–14 yr <14 or >25; adults: [age 14 or older] <11 or >24); depth of breathing (adults V_T 500 ml at rest, infants 6–8 ml/kg); timing ratio; decreased vital capacity

Cardiac output, decreased

Definition: inadequate blood pumped by heart to meet the metabolic demands of the body

Related factors: altered heart rate/rhythm; altered stroke volume; altered preload, altered afterload, altered contractility

Defining characteristics:

Altered heart rate/rhythm: arrhythmias (tachycardia, bradycardia); palpitations; EKG changes

Altered preload: jugular vein distention; fatigue; edema; murmurs; increased/decreased central venous pressure (CVP); increased/decreased pulmonary artery wedge pressure (PAWP); weight gain

Altered afterload: cold/clammy skin; shortness of breath/dyspnea; oliguria; prolonged capillary refill; decreased peripheral pulses; variations in blood pressure readings; increased/decreased systemic vascular resistance (SVR); increased/decreased pulmonary vascular resistance (PVR); skin color changes

Altered contractility: crackles; cough; orthopnea/paroxysmal nocturnal dyspnea; cardiac output < 4 L/min; cardiac index < 2.5 L/min; decreased ejection fraction, Stroke Volume Index (SVI), Left Ventricular Stroke Work Index (LVSWI); S3 or S4 sounds

Behavioral/emotional: anxiety; restlessness

Caregiver role strain

Definition: difficulty in performing a family caregiver role

Related factors:

Resources: caregiver is not developmentally ready for caregiver role; lack of caregiver privacy; lack of support; insufficient time; inadequate transportation; insufficient finances; inadequate equipment for providing care; inadequate community resources (e.g., respite services, recreational resources); inadequate physical environment for providing care (e.g., housing, temperature, safety); inexperience with caregiving; lack of knowledge about or difficulty accessing community resources; emotional strength; physical energy; assistance and support (formal and informal)

Caregiver-care receiver relationship: history of poor relationship; presence of abuse or violence; unrealistic expectations of caregiver by care receiver; mental status of elder inhibiting conversation

Family processes: history of marginal family coping; history of family dysfunction

Care receiver health status: illness severity; illness chronicity; increasing care needs/dependency; unpredictability of illness course; instability of care receiver's health; problem behaviors; psychological or cognitive problems; addiction or codependency

Caregiving activities: amount of activities; complexity of activities; 24-hour care responsibilities; ongoing changes in activities; discharge of family members to home with significant care needs; years of caregiving; unpredictability of care situation

Caregiver health status: physical problems; psychological or cognitive problems; addiction of codependency; marginal coping patterns; unrealistic expectations of self; inability to fulfill one's own or other's expectations

Socioeconomic: isolation from others; competing role commitments; alienation from family, friends, and co-workers; insufficient recreation

Defining characteristics:
Caregiving activities: difficulty performing/completing tasks; preoccupation with care routine; apprehension about the future regarding care receiver's health and the caregiver's ability to provide care; apprehension about care receiver's care if caregiver becomes ill or dies; dysfunctional change in caregiving activities; apprehension about possible institutionalization of care receiver
Caregiver health status:

- *Physical:* GI upset (e.g., mild stomach cramps, vomiting, diarrhea, recurrent gastric ulcer episodes); weight change; rash; hypertension; cardiovascular disease; diabetes; fatigue; headaches
- *Emotional:* impaired individual coping; feeling depressed; disturbed sleep; anger; stress; increased nervousness; increased emotional lability; impatience; lack of time to meet personal needs; frustration
- *Socioeconomic:* withdraws from social life; changes in leisure activities; low work productivity; refuses career advancement

Caregiver-care receiver relationship: grief/uncertainty regarding changed relationship with care receiver; difficulty watching care receiver go through the illness
Family processes: family conflict; concerns about family members

Caregiver role strain, risk for

Definition: caregiver is vulnerable for felt difficulty in performing the family caregiver role
Risk factors: caregiver is not developmentally ready for caregiver role (e.g., a young adult needing to provide care for middle-aged person); inadequate physical environment for providing care (e.g., housing, transportation, community services, equipment); unpredictable illness course or instability in the care receiver's health; psychological or cognitive problems in care receiver; presence of situational stressors which normally affect families (e.g., significant loss, disaster or crisis, economic vulnerability, major life events); presence of abuse or violence; premature birth/congenital defect; past history of poor relationship between caregiver and care receiver; marginal family adaptation or dysfunction prior to the caregiving situation; marginal caregiver's coping patterns; lack of respite and recreation for caregiver; inexperience with caregiving; caregiver is female; addiction or codependency; care receiver exhibits deviant, bizarre behavior; caregiver's competing role commitments; caregiver health impairment; illness severity of the care receiver; caregiver is spouse; complexity/amount of caregiving tasks; developmental delay or retardation of the care receiver or caregiver; discharge of family member with significant home care needs; duration of caregiving required; family/caregiver isolation

Communication, impaired verbal

Definition: decreased, delayed, or absent ability to receive, process, transmit, and use a system of symbols
Related factors: decrease in circulation to brain; cultural difference; psychological barriers (e.g., psychosis, lack of stimuli); physical barrier (e.g., tracheostomy, intubation); anatomical defect (e.g., cleft palate, alteration of the neuromuscular visual system, auditory system, or phonatory apparatus); brain tumor; differences related to developmental age; side-effects of medication; environmental barriers; absence of significant others; altered perceptions; lack of information; stress; alteration of self-esteem or self-concept; physiological conditions; alteration of central nervous system; weakening of the musculoskeletal system; emotional conditions
Defining characteristics: willful refusal to speak; disorientation in the three spheres of time, space, person; unable to speak dominant language; does not or cannot speak; speaks or verbalizes with difficulty;

inappropriate verbalization; difficulty forming words or sentences (e.g., aphonia, dyslalia, dysarthria); stuttering; slurring; difficulty expressing thought verbally (e.g., aphasia, dysphasia apraxia, dyslexia); dyspnea; absence of eye contact or difficulty in selective attending; difficulty in comprehending and maintaining the usual communication pattern; partial or total visual deficit; inability or difficulty in use of facial or body expressions

Communication, readiness for enhanced

Definition: a pattern of exchanging information and ideas with others that is sufficient for meeting one's needs and life's goals and can be strengthened

Defining characteristics: expresses willingness to enhance communication; able to speak or write a language; forms words, phrases, and language; expresses thoughts and feelings; uses and interprets non-verbal cues appropriately; expresses satisfaction with ability to share information and ideas with others

Conflict, decisional (specify)

Definition: uncertainty about course of action to be taken when choice among competing actions involves risk, loss, or challenge to personal life values

Related factors: support system deficit; perceived threat to value system; multiple or divergent sources of information; lack of relevant information; unclear personal values/beliefs

Defining characteristics: lack of experience or interference with decision making; verbalization of undesired consequences of alternative actions being considered; verbalized uncertainty about choice; vacillation between alternative choices; delayed decision making; verbalized feeling of distress while attempting a decision; self-focusing; physical signs of distress or tension (e.g., increased heart rate, increased muscle tension, restlessness); questioning personal values and beliefs while attempting a decision

Conflict, parental role

Definition: parent experience(s) of role confusion and conflict in response to crisis

Related factors: change in marital status; home care of a child with special needs (e.g., apnea monitoring, postural drainage, hyperalimentation); interruptions of family life due to home care regime (e.g., treatments, caregivers, lack of respite); specialized care centers, policies; separation from child due to chronic illness; intimidation with invasive or restrictive modalities (e.g., isolation, intubation), specialized care centers, policies

Defining characteristics: parent(s) express concern(s) about changes in parental role, family functioning, family communication, family health, parent(s) expresses concern(s)/feeling(s) of inadequacy to provide for child's physical and emotional needs during hospitalization or in home; demonstrated disruption in care taking routines; expresses concern about perceived loss of control over decisions relating to their child; reluctant to participate in usual care-taking activities even with encouragement and support; verbalizes or demonstrates feelings of guilt, anger, fear, anxiety and/or frustrations about effect of child's illness on family process

Confusion, acute

Definition: abrupt onset of a cluster of global, transient changes and disturbances in attention, cognition, psychomotor activity, level of consciousness, and/or sleep/wake cycle

Related factors: over 60 years of age; alcohol abuse; delirium; dementia; drug abuse
Defining characteristics: lack of motivation to initiate and/or follow through with goal-directed or purposeful behavior; fluctuation in psychomotor activity; misperceptions; fluctuation in cognition; increased agitation or restlessness; fluctuation in level of consciousness; fluctuation in sleep-wake cycle; hallucinations

Confusion, chronic

Definition: irreversible, long-standing and/or progressive deterioration of intellect and personality characterized by decreased ability to interpret environmental stimuli, decreased capacity for intellectual thought processes and manifested by disturbances of memory, orientation, and behavior
Related factors: multi-infarct dementia; Korsakoff's psychosis; head injury; Alzheimer's disease; cerebral vascular accident
Defining characteristics: altered interpretation/response to stimuli; clinical evidence of organic impairment; progressive/long-standing cognitive impairment; altered personality; impaired memory (short-term and long-term); impaired socialization, no change in level of consciousness

Constipation

Definition: decrease in normal frequency of defecation accompanied by difficult or incomplete passage of stool and/or passage of excessively hard, dry stool
Related factors:
Functional: recent environmental changes; habitual denial/ignoring of urge to defecate; insufficient physical activity; irregular defecation habits; inadequate toileting (e.g., timeliness, positioning for defecation, privacy); abdominal muscle weakness
Psychological: depression; emotional stress; mental confusion
Pharmacological: antilipemic agents; laxative overdose; calcium carbonate; aluminum-containing antacids; nonsteroidal anti-inflammatory agents; opiates; anticholinergics; diuretics; iron salts; phenothiazides; sedatives; sympathomimetics; bismuth salts; antidepressants; calcium channel blockers
Mechanical: rectal abscess or ulcer; pregnancy; rectal anal fissures; tumors; megacolon (Hirschsprung's disease); electrolyte imbalance; rectal prolapse; prostate enlargement; neurological impairment; rectal anal stricture; rectocele; postsurgical obstruction; hemorrhoids; obesity
Physiological: poor eating habits; decreased motility of gastrointestinal tract; inadequate dentition or oral hygiene; insufficient fiber intake; insufficient fluid intake; change in usual foods and eating patterns; dehydration
Defining characteristics: change in bowel pattern; bright red blood with stool; presence of soft, paste-like stool in rectum; distended abdomen; dark, black, or tarry stool; increased abdominal pressure; percussed abdominal dullness; pain with defecation; decreased volume of stool; straining with defecation; decreased frequency; dry, hard, formed stool; palpable rectal mass; feeling of rectal fullness or pressure; abdominal pain; unable to pass stool; anorexia; headache; change in abdominal growling (borborygmi); indigestion; atypical presentations in older adults (e.g., change in mental status, urinary incontinence, unexplained falls, elevated body temperature); severe flatus; generalized fatigue; hypoactive or hyperactive bowel sounds; palpable abdominal mass; abdominal tenderness with or without palpable muscle resistance; nausea and/or vomiting; oozing liquid stool

Constipation, perceived

Definition: self-diagnosis of constipation and abuse of laxatives, enemas, and suppositories to ensure a daily bowel movement

Related factors: impaired thought processes; faulty appraisal; cultural/family health beliefs

Defining characteristics: expectation of a daily bowel movement with the resulting overuse of laxatives, enemas, and suppositories; expectation of passage of stool at same time every day

Constipation, risk for

Definition: at risk for a decrease in a person's normal frequency of defecation accompanied by difficult or incomplete passage of stool and/or passage of excessively hard, dry stool

Risk factors:

Functional: habitual denial/ignoring of urge to defecate; recent environmental changes; inadequate toileting (e.g., timeliness, positioning for defecation, privacy); irregular defecation habits; insufficient physical activity; abdominal muscle weakness

Psychological: emotional stress; mental confusion; depression

Physiological: insufficient fiber intake; dehydration; inadequate dentition or oral hygiene; poor eating habits; insufficient fluid intake; change in usual foods and eating patterns; decreased motility of gastrointestinal tract

Pharmacological: phenothiazides, nonsteroidal anti-inflammatory agents; sedatives; aluminum-containing antacids; laxative overuse; iron salts; anticholinergics; antidepressants; anticonvulsants; antilipemic agents; calcium channel blockers; calcium carbonate; diuretics; sympathomimetics; opiates; bismuth salts

Mechanical: rectal abscess or ulcer; pregnancy; rectal anal stricture; postsurgical obstruction; rectal anal fissures; megacolon (Hirschsprung's disease); electrolyte imbalance; tumors; prostate enlargement; rectocele; rectal prolapse; neurological impairment; hemorrhoids; obesity

Coping, ineffective community

Definition: a pattern of community activities for adaptation and problem solving that is unsatisfactory for meeting the demands or needs of the community

Related factors: natural or man-made disasters; ineffective or nonexistent community systems (e.g., lack of emergency medical system, transportation system, or disaster planning systems); deficits in community social support services and resources; inadequate resources for problem solving

Defining characteristics: expressed community powerlessness; deficits of community participation; excessive community conflicts; expressed vulnerability; high illness rates; stressors perceived as excessive; community does not meet its own expectations; increased social problems (e.g., homicides, vandalism, arson, terrorism, robbery, infanticide, abuse, divorce, unemployment, poverty, militancy, mental illness)

Coping, readiness for enhanced community

Definition: a pattern of cognitive and behavioral efforts to manage demands that is sufficient for well-being and can be strengthened

Defining characteristics: defines stressors as manageable; seeks social support; uses a broad range of problem-oriented and emotion-oriented strategies; uses spiritual resources; acknowledges power; seeks knowledge of new strategies; is aware of possible environmental changes

Coping, defensive

Definition: repeated projection of falsely positive self-evaluation based on a self-protective pattern that defends against underlying perceived threats to positive self-regard

Related factors: to be developed

Defining characteristics: grandiosity; rationalizes failures; hypersensitive to slight/criticism; denial of obvious problems/weaknesses; projection of blame/responsibility; lack of follow through or participation in treatment or therapy; superior attitude toward others; hostile laughter or ridicule of others; difficulty in reality-testing perceptions; difficulty establishing/maintaining relationships

Coping, ineffective

Definition: inability to form a valid appraisal of the stressors, inadequate choices of practiced responses, and/or inability to use available resources

Related factors: gender differences in coping strategies; inadequate level of confidence in ability to cope; uncertainty; inadequate social support created by characteristics of relationships; inadequate level of perception of control; inadequate resources available; high degree of threat; situational or maturational crisis; disturbance in pattern of tension release; inadequate opportunity to prepare for stressor; inability to conserve adaptive energies; disturbance in pattern of appraisal of threat

Defining characteristics: lack of goal-directed behavior/resolution of problem, including inability to attend to and difficulty organizing information; sleep disturbance; abuse of chemical agents; decreased use of social support; use of forms of coping that impede adaptive behavior; poor concentration; fatigue; inadequate problem solving; verbalization of inability to cope or inability to ask for help; inability to meet basic needs; destructive behavior toward self or others; inability to meet role expectations; high illness rate; change in usual communication patterns; risk taking

Coping, readiness for enhanced

Definition: a pattern of cognitive and behavioral efforts to manage demands that is sufficient for well-being and can be strengthened

Defining characteristics: defines stressors as manageable; seeks social support; uses a broad range of problem-oriented and emotional-oriented strategies; uses spiritual resources; acknowledges power

Coping, compromised family

Definition: usually supportive primary person (family member or close friend) provides insufficient, ineffective or compromised support, comfort assistance or encouragement that may be needed by the client to manage or master adaptive tasks related to his/her health challenge

Related factors: temporary preoccupation by a significant person who is trying to manage emotional conflicts and personal suffering and is unable to perceive or act effectively in regard to client's needs; temporary family disorganization and role changes; prolonged disease or disability progression that exhausts supportive capacity of significant people; other situational or developmental crises or situations the significant person may be facing; inadequate or incorrect information or understanding by a primary person; little support provided by client, in turn, for primary person

Defining characteristics:

Objective: significant person attempts assistive or supportive behaviors with less than satisfactory results; significant person displays protective behavior disproportionate (too little or too much) to the client's abilities or need for autonomy; significant person withdraws or enters into limited or temporary personal communication with the client at the time of need

Subjective: client expresses or confirms a concern or complaint about significant other's response to his or her health problem; significant person describes or confirms an inadequate understanding or knowledge base, which interferes with effective assistive or supportive behaviors; significant person describes preoccupation with personal reaction (e.g., fear, anticipatory grief, guilt, anxiety) to client's illness, disability, or other situational or developmental crises

Coping, disabled family

Definition: behavior of significant person (family member or other primary person) that disables his/her capacities and the client's capacities to effectively address tasks essential to either person's adaptation to the health challenge

Related factors: significant person with chronically unexpressed feelings of guilt, anxiety, hostility, despair, etc., arbitrary handling of family's resistance to treatment, which tends to solidify defensiveness as it fails to deal adequately with underlying anxiety; dissonant discrepancy of coping styles for dealing with adaptive tasks by the significant person and client or among significant people; highly ambivalent family relationships

Defining characteristics: intolerance; agitation; depression; aggression; hostility; taking on illness signs of client; rejection; psychosomaticism; neglectful care of the client in regard to basic human needs and/or illness treatment; impaired restructuring of a meaningful life for self; impaired individualization; prolonged over-concern for client; distortion of reality regarding the client's health problem, including extreme denial about its existence or severity; desertion; decisions and actions by family that are detrimental to economic or social well-being; carrying on usual routines, disregarding client's needs; abandonment; client's development of helplessness, inactive dependence; disregarding needs

Coping, readiness for enhanced family

Definition: effective managing of adaptive tasks by family member involved with the client's health challenge, who now exhibits desire and readiness for enhanced health and growth in regard to self and in relation to the client

Related factors: needs sufficiently gratified and adaptive tasks effectively addressed to enable goals of self-actualization to surface

Defining characteristics: individual expressing interest in making contact on a one-to-one basis or on a mutual-aid group basis with another person who has experienced a similar situation; family member moving in direction of health promoting and enriching life-style that supports and monitors maturational processes, audits and negotiates treatment programs, and chooses experiences that optimize wellness; family member attempting to describe growth impact of crisis on his or her own values, priorities, goal, or relationships

Death syndrome, risk for sudden infant

Definition: presence of risk factors for sudden death of an infant under one year of age

Risk factors:

Modifiable: infants placed to sleep in the prone or side-lying position; prenatal and/or postnatal infant smoke exposure; infant over-heating/over-wrapping; soft under-layment/loose articles in the sleep environment; delayed or nonattendance of prenatal care

Potentially modifiable: low birth weight; prematurity; young maternal age
Nonmodifiable: male gender; ethnicity (e.g., African American or Native American race of mother); seasonality of Sudden Infant Death Syndrome (SIDS) deaths (higher in winter and fall months); SIDS mortality peaks between infant age of two to four months

Denial, ineffective
Definition: conscious or unconscious attempt to disavow the knowledge or meaning of an event to reduce anxiety/fear, but to the detriment of health
Related factors: to be developed
Defining characteristics: delays seeking or refuses health care attention to the detriment of health; does not perceive personal relevance of symptoms or danger; displaces source of symptoms to other organs; displays inappropriate affect; does not admit fear of death or invalidism; makes dismissive gestures or comments when speaking of distressing events; minimizes symptoms; unable to admit impact of disease on life pattern; uses home remedies (self-treatment) to relieve symptoms; displaces fear of impact of the condition

Dentition, impaired
Definition: disruption in tooth development/eruption patterns or structural integrity of individual teeth
Related factors: ineffective oral hygiene; sensitivity to heat or cold; barriers to self-care; access or economic barriers to professional care; nutritional deficits; dietary habits; genetic predisposition; selected prescription medications; premature loss of primary teeth; excessive intake of fluorides; chronic vomiting; chronic use of tobacco, coffee, tea, or red wine; lack of knowledge regarding dental health; excessive use of abrasive cleaning agents; bruxism
Defining characteristics: excessive plaque; crown or root caries; halitosis; tooth enamel discoloration; toothache; loose teeth; excessive calculus; incomplete eruption for age (may be primary or permanent teeth); malocclusion or tooth misalignment; premature loss of primary teeth; worn down or abraded teeth; tooth fracture(s); missing teeth or complete absence; erosion of enamel; asymmetrical facial expression

Development, risk for altered
Definition: at risk for delay of 25% or more in one or more of the areas of social or self-regulatory behavior, or cognitive, language, gross or fine motor skills
Risk factors:
Prenatal: maternal age <15 or >35 years; substance abuse; infections; genetic or endocrine disorders; unplanned or unwanted pregnancy; lack of, late, or poor prenatal care; inadequate nutrition; illiteracy; poverty
Individual: prematurity; seizures; congenital or genetic disorders; positive drug screening test; brain damage (e.g., hemorrhage in postnatal period, shaken baby, abuse, accident); vision impairment; hearing impairment or frequent otitis media; chronic illness; technology-dependent; failure to thrive, inadequate nutrition; foster or adopted child; lead poisoning; chemotherapy; radiation therapy; natural disaster; behavior disorders; substance abuse
Environmental: poverty; violence
Caregiver: abuse; mental illness; mental retardation or severe learning disability

Diarrhea
Definition: passage of loose, unformed stools
Related factors:
Psychological: high stress levels and anxiety
Situational: alcohol abuse; toxins; laxative abuse; radiation; tube feedings; adverse effects of medications; contaminants; travel
Physiological: inflammation; malabsorption; infectious processes; irritation; parasites
Defining characteristics: hyperactive bowel sounds; at least three loose liquid stools per day; urgency; abdominal pain; cramping

Disuse syndrome, risk for
Definition: at risk for deterioration of body systems as the result of prescribed or unavoidable musculoskeletal inactivity
Risk factors: severe pain; mechanical immobilization; altered level of consciousness; prescribed immobilization; paralysis
Note: Complications from immobility can include pressure ulcer, constipation, stasis of pulmonary secretions, thrombosis, urinary tract infection and/or retention, decreased strength or endurance, orthostatic hypotension, decreased range of joint motion, disorientation, body-image disturbance, and powerlessness.

Diversional activity deficient
Definition: decreased stimulation from (or interest or engagement in) recreational or leisure activities
Related factors: environmental lack of diversional activity as in long-term hospitalization; frequent, lengthy treatments
Defining characteristics: usual hobbies cannot be undertaken in hospital; patient's statements regarding: boredom, wish there was something to do, to read, etc.

Energy field disturbance
Definition: disruption of the flow of energy surrounding a person's being results in disharmony of the body, mind, and/or spirit
Related factors: slowing or blocking of energy flows secondary to:
Pathophysiologic: illness (specify); pregnancy; injury
Treatment-related: immobility; labor and delivery; perioperative experience; chemotherapy
Situational (personal, environmental): pain; fear; anxiety; grieving; maturational factors; age-related developmental difficulties or crisis (specify)
Defining characteristics: perceptions of changes in patterns of energy flow, such as: movement (wave, spike, tingling, dense, flowing, sounds [tone, words]) temperature change (warmth, coolness); visual changes (image, color); disruption of the field (deficit, hole, spike, bulge, obstruction, congestion, diminished flow in energy field)

Environmental interpretation syndrome, impaired
Definition: consistent lack of orientation to person, place, time, or circumstances over more than three to six months, necessitating a protective environment

Related factors: depression; Huntington's disease; dementia (e.g., Alzheimer's, multi-infarct dementia, Pick's disease, AIDS dementia, alcoholism, Parkinson's disease)

Defining characteristics: chronic confusional states; consistent disorientation in known and unknown environments; loss of occupation or social functioning from memory decline; slow in responding to questions; inability to follow simple directions, instructions; inability to concentrate; inability to reason

Failure to thrive, adult

Definition: progressive functional deterioration of a physical and cognitive nature; the individual's ability to live with multisystem diseases, cope with ensuing problems, and manage his/her care are remarkably diminished

Related factors: depression; apathy; fatigue

Defining characteristics: anorexia—does not eat meals when offered; states does not have an appetite, not hungry, or "I don't want to eat"; inadequate nutritional intake—eating less than body requirements; consumes minimal to none of food at most meals (i.e., consumes less than 75% of normal requirements at each or most meals); weight loss (decreased body mass from base line weight)—5% unintentional weight loss in 1 month, 10% unintentional weight loss in six months; physical decline (decline in bodily function)—evidence of fatigue, dehydration, incontinence of bowel and bladder; frequent exacerbation of chronic health problems such as pneumonia or urinary tract infections; cognitive decline (decline in mental processing)—as evidenced by problems with responding appropriately to environmental stimuli, demonstrates difficulty in reasoning, decision making, judgment, memory and concentration, decreased perception; decreased social skills/social withdrawal—noticeable decrease from usual past behavior in attempts to form or participate in cooperative and interdependent relationships (e.g., decreased verbal communication with staff, family, friends); decreased participation in activities of daily living that the older person once enjoyed; self-care deficit—no longer looks after or takes charge of physical cleanliness or appearance; difficulty performing simple self-care tasks; neglects home environment; altered mood state—expresses loss of interest in pleasurable outlets such as food, sex, work, friends, family, hobbies, or entertainment; verbalizes desire for death

Falls, risk for

Definition: increased susceptibility to falling that may cause physical harm

Risk factors:

Adults: history of falls; wheelchair use; age 65 or over; female (if elderly); lives alone; lower limb prosthesis; use of assistive devices (e.g., walker, cane)

Physiological: presence of acute illness; postoperative conditions; visual difficulties; hearing difficulties; arthritis; orthostatic hypotension; sleeplessness; faintness when turning or extending neck; anemias; vascular disease; neoplasms (i.e., fatigue/limited mobility); urgency and/or incontinence; diarrhea; decreased lower extremity strength; postprandial blood sugar changes; foot problems; impaired physical mobility; impaired balance; difficulty with gait; proprioceptive deficits (e.g., unilateral neglect); neuropathy

Cognitive: diminished mental status (e.g., confusion, delirium, dementia, impaired reality testing)

Medications: antihypertensive agents; Angiotensin-converting Enzyme (ACE) inhibitors; diuretics; tricyclic antidepressants; alcohol use; antianxiety agents; narcotics; hypnotics or tranquilizers

Environment: restraints; weather conditions (e.g., wet floors/ice); throw/scatter rugs; cluttered environment; unfamiliar, dimly lit room; no antislip material in bath and/or shower

Children: < two years of age; male gender when < one year of age; lack of auto restraints; lack of gate on stairs; lack of window guard; bed located near window; unattended infant on bed/changing table/sofa; lack of parental supervision

Family processes, dysfunctional, alcoholism

Definition: psychosocial, spiritual, and physiological functions of the family unit are chronically disorganized, leading to conflict, denial of problems, resistance to change, ineffective problem-solving, and a series of self-perpetuating crises

Related factors: abuse of alcohol; genetic predisposition; lack of problem-solving skills; inadequate coping skills; family history of alcoholism, resistance to treatment; biochemical influences; addictive personality

Defining characteristics:

Roles and relationships: inconsistent parenting/low perception of parental support; ineffective spouse communication/marital problems; intimacy dysfunction; deterioration in family relationships/disturbed family dynamics; altered role function/disruption of family roles; closed communication systems; chronic family problems; family denial; lack of cohesiveness; neglected obligations; lack of skills necessary for relationships; reduced ability of family members to relate to each other for mutual growth and maturation; family unable to meet security needs of its members; disrupted family rituals; economic problems; family does not demonstrate respect for individuality and autonomy of its members; triangulating of family relationships; pattern of rejection

Behavioral: refusal to get help/inability to accept and receive help appropriately; inadequate understanding or knowledge of alcoholism; ineffective problem-solving skills; loss of control of drinking; manipulation; rationalization/denial of problems; blaming; inability to meet emotional needs of its members; alcohol abuse; broken promises; criticizing; dependency; impaired communication; difficulty with intimate relationships; enabling to maintain drinking; expression of anger inappropriately; isolation; inability to meet spiritual needs of its members; inability to express or accept wide range of feelings; inability to deal with traumatic experiences constructively; inability to adapt to change; immaturity; harsh self-judgment; lying; lack of dealing with conflict; lack of reliability; nicotine addiction; orientation toward tension relief rather than achievement of goals; seeking approval and affirmation; difficulty having fun; agitation; chaos; contradictory, paradoxical communication; diminished physical contact; disturbances in academic performance in children; disturbances in concentration; escalating conflict, failure to accomplish current or past developmental tasks; difficulty with life cycle transitions; family special occasions are alcohol centered; controlling communication/power struggles; self-blaming; stress-related physical illnesses; substance abuse other than alcohol; unresolved grief; verbal abuse of spouse or parent

Feelings: insecurity; lingering resentment; mistrust; vulnerability; rejection; repressed emotions; responsibility for alcoholic's behavior; shame/embarrassment; unhappiness; powerlessness; anger/suppressed rage; anxiety or tension or distress; emotional isolation/loneliness; frustration; guilt; hopelessness; hurt; decreased self-esteem/worthlessness; hostility; lack of identify; fear; loss; emotional control by others; misunderstood; moodiness; abandonment; being different from other people; being unloved; confused love and pity; confusion; failure; depression; dissatisfaction

Family processes, interrupted
Definition: change in family relationships and/or functioning
Related factors: power shift of family members; family roles shift; shift in health status of a family member; developmental transition and/or crisis; situation transition and/or crisis; informal or formal interaction with community; modification in family social status; modification in family finances
Defining characteristics: changes in: power alliances, assigned tasks, effectiveness in completing assigned tasks, mutual support, availability for affective responsiveness and intimacy, patterns and rituals, participation in problem solving, participation in decision-making, communication patterns, availability for emotional support, satisfaction with family, stress-reduction behaviors, expressions of conflict with and/or isolation form community resources, somatic complaints, expressions of conflict within family

Family processes, readiness for enhanced
Definition: a pattern of family functioning that is sufficient to support the well-being of family members and can be strengthened
Defining characteristics: expresses willingness to enhance family dynamics; family functioning meets physical, social, and psychological needs of family members; activities support the safety and growth of family members; communication is adequate; relationships are generally positive; interdependent with community; family task(s) are accomplished; family roles are flexible and appropriate for developmental stages; respect for family members is evident; family adapts to change; boundaries of family members are maintained; energy level of family supports activities of daily living; balance exists between autonomy and cohesiveness

Fatigue
Definition: an overwhelming sustained sense of exhaustion and decreased capacity for physical and mental work at usual level
Related factors:
Psychological: boring lifestyle; stress; anxiety; depression
Environmental: humidity; lights; noise; temperature
Situational: negative life events; occupation
Physiological: sleep deprivation; pregnancy; poor physical condition; disease states; increased physical exertion; malnutrition; anemia
Defining characteristics: inability to restore energy even after sleep; lack of energy or inability to maintain usual level of physical activity; increase in rest requirements; tired; inability to maintain usual routines; verbalization of an unremitting and overwhelming lack of energy; lethargic or listless; perceived need for additional energy to accomplish routine tasks; increase in physical complaints; compromised concentration; disinterest in surroundings, introspection; decreased performance; compromised libido; drowsy; feelings of guilt for not keeping up with responsibilities

Fear
Definition: response to perceived threat that is consciously recognized as a danger
Related factors: phobic stimulus; separation from support system in potentially stressful situation (e.g., hospitalization, hospital procedures); natural/innate origin (e.g., sudden noise, height, pain, loss

of physical support); learned response (e.g., conditioning, modeling from or identification with others); unfamiliarity with environmental experiences; language barrier; sensory impairment; innate releasers (neurotransmitters)

Defining characteristics: report of: apprehension, increased tension, decreased self-assurance, excitement, being scared, jitteriness, dread, alarm, terror, panic

Cognitive: identifies object of fear; stimulus believed to be a threat; diminished productivity, learning ability, problem-solving ability

Behaviors: increased alertness; avoidance or attack behaviors; impulsiveness; narrowed focus on "it" (i.e., the focus of the fear)

Physiological: increased pulse; anorexia; nausea; vomiting; diarrhea; muscle tightness; fatigue; increased respiratory rate and shortness of breath; pallor; increased perspiration; increased systolic blood pressure; pupil dilation; dry mouth

Fluid balance, readiness for enhanced

Definition: a pattern of equilibrium between fluid volume and chemical composition of body fluids that is sufficient for meeting physical needs and can be strengthened

Defining characteristics: expresses willingness to enhance fluid balance; stable weight; moist mucous membranes; food and fluid intake adequate for daily needs; straw-colored urine with specific gravity within normal limits; good tissue turgor; no excessive thirst; urine output appropriate for intake; no evidence of edema or dehydration

Fluid volume, deficient

Definition: decreased intravascular, interstitial and/or intracellular fluid. This refers to dehydration, water loss alone without change in sodium.

Related factors: active fluid volume loss; failure of regulatory mechanisms

Defining characteristics: decreased urine output; increased urine concentration; weakness; sudden weight loss (except in third-spacing); decreased venous filling; increased body temperature; decreased pulse volume/pressure; change in mental state; elevated hematocrit; decreased skin/tongue turgor; dry skin/mucous membranes; thirst; increased pulse rate; decreased blood pressure

Fluid volume deficient, risk for

Definition: at risk of experiencing vascular, cellular, or intracellular dehydration

Risk factors: factors influencing fluids needs (e.g., hypermetabolic state); medication (e.g., diuretics); loss of fluid through abnormal routes (e.g., indwelling tubes); knowledge deficiency related to fluid volume; extremes of age; deviations affecting access to or intake or absorption of fluids (e.g., physical immobility); extremes of weight; excessive losses through normal routes (e.g., diarrhea)

Fluid volume, excess

Definition: increased isotonic fluid retention

Related factors: compromised regulatory mechanism; excess fluid intake; excess sodium intake

Defining characteristics: jugular vein distention; decreased hemoglobin and hematocrit; weight gain over short period; dyspnea or shortness of breath; intake exceeds output; pleural effusion; orthopnea;

S₃ heart sound; pulmonary artery pressure changes; oliguria; specific gravity changes; azotemia; altered electrolytes; restlessness; anxiety; anasarca; abnormal breath sounds (rales or crackles); edema; increased central venous pressure; positive hepatojugular reflex

Fluid volume, risk for imbalanced

Definition: at risk for a decrease, increase, or rapid shift from one to the other of intravascular, interstitial, and/or intracellular fluid. This refers to body fluid loss, gain, or both.

Risk factors: scheduled for major invasive procedures; other risk factors to be determined

Gas exchange, impaired

Definition: excess or deficit in oxygenation and/or carbon dioxide elimination at the alveolar-capillary membrane

Related factors: ventilation perfusion imbalance; alveolar-capillary membrane changes

Defining characteristics: visual disturbances; decreased carbon dioxide; tachycardia; hypercapnia; restlessness; somnolence; irritability; hypoxia; confusion; dyspnea; abnormal arterial blood gases; cyanosis (in neonates, only); abnormal skin color (pale, dusky); hypoxemia; hypercarbia; headache upon awakening; abnormal rate, rhythm, depth of breathing; diaphoresis; abnormal arterial pH; nasal flaring

Grieving, anticipatory

Definition: intellectual and emotional responses and behaviors by which individuals, families, communities work through the process of modifying self-concept based on the perception of potential loss

Related factors: to be developed; possible non-NANDA factors: impending death; possible loss of body part or function; potential loss of significant person, possession, animal; potential loss (specify)

Defining characteristics: expressions of distress at potential loss; sorrow; guilt; denial of potential loss; anger; altered communication patterns; potential loss of significant object; denial of the significance of the loss; bargaining; alteration in eating habits, sleep patterns, dream patterns, activity level, libido; difficulty taking on new or different roles; resolution of grief prior to the reality of loss

Grieving, dysfunctional

Definition: extended, unsuccessful use of intellectual and emotional responses by which individuals, families, communities attempt to work through the process of modifying self-concept based upon the perception of loss

Related factors:

General: preloss neuroticism; preloss psychological symptoms; frequency of major life events; predisposition for anxiety and feelings of inadequacy; past psychiatric or mental health treatment

Perinatal: later gestational age at time of loss; limited time since perinatal loss and subsequent conception; length of life of infant; absence of other living children; congential anomaly; number of past perinatal losses; martial adjustment problems; viewing of ultrasound images of the fetus

Defining characteristics: persistent anxiety; depression; altered activities of daily living; prolonged difficulty coping; loss-associated sense of despair; intrusive images; feelings of inadequacy; decreased self-esteem; diminished sense of control; dependency; death anxiety; self-criticism

Grieving, risk for dysfunctional
Definition: at risk for extended, unsuccessful use of intellectual and emotional responses and behaviors by an individual, family, or community following a death or perception of loss
Risk factors:
General: preloss neuroticism; preloss psychological symptoms; frequency of major life events; predisposition for anxiety and feelings of inadequacy; past psychiatric or mental health treatment
Perinatal: later gestational age at time of loss; limited time since perinatal loss and subsequent conception; length of life of infant; absence of other living children; congenital anomaly; number of past perinatal losses; marital adjustment problems; viewing of ultrasound images of the fetus

Growth and development, delayed
Definition: deviations from age group norms
Related factors: prescribed dependence; indifference; separation from significant others; environmental and stimulation deficiencies; effects of physical disability; inadequate care-taking; inconsistent responsiveness; multiple caretakers
Defining characteristics: altered physical growth; delay or difficulty in performing skills (motor, social, expressive) typical of age group; inability to perform self-care or self-control activities appropriate for age; flat affect; listlessness, decreased responses

Growth, risk for disproportionate
Definition: at risk for growth above the 97th percentile or below the third percentile for age, crossing two percentile channels; disproportionate growth
Risk factors:
Prenatal: congenital/genetic disorders; maternal nutrition; multiple gestation; teratogen exposure; substance use/abuse
Individual: infection; prematurity; malnutrition; organic and inorganic factors; caregiver and/or individual maladaptive feeding behaviors; anorexia; insatiable appetite; chronic illness; substance abuse
Environmental: deprivation; teratogen exposure; lead poisoning; poverty; violence; natural disasters
Caregiver: abuse; mental illness; mental retardation; severe learning disability

Health maintenance, ineffective
Definition: inability to identify, manage and/or seek out help to maintain health
Related factors: ineffective individual or family coping; perceptual/cognitive impairment (complete/partial lack of gross and/or fine motor skills); lack of, or significant alteration in communication skills (written, verbal and/or gestural); unachieved developmental tasks; lack of material resources; dysfunctional grieving; disabling spiritual distress; lack of ability to make deliberate and thoughtful judgments

Defining characteristics: history of lack of health-seeking behavior; reported or observed lack of equipment, financial and/or other resources; reported or observed impairment of personal support systems; expressed interest in improving health behaviors; demonstrated lack of knowledge regarding basic health practices; demonstrated lack of adaptive behaviors to internal/external environmental changes; reported or observed inability to take responsibility for meeting basic health practices in any or all functional pattern areas

Health-seeking behaviors (specify)
Definition: active seeking (by a person in stable health) of ways to alter personal health habits and/or the environment in order to move toward a higher level of health
Related factors: to be developed
Defining characteristics: expressed or observed desire to seek a higher level of wellness; demonstrated or observed lack of knowledge in health-promotion behaviors; stated or observed unfamiliarity with wellness community resources; expression of concern about current environmental conditions on health status; expressed or observed desire for increased control of health practice
Note: Stable health is defined as achievement of age-appropriate illness-prevention measures; client reports good or excellent health, and signs and symptoms of disease, if present, are controlled.

Home maintenance, impaired
Definition: inability to independently maintain a safe growth-promoting immediate environment
Related factors: individual/family member disease or injury; unfamiliarity with neighborhood resources; lack of role modeling; lack of knowledge; insufficient family organization or planning; inadequate support systems; impaired cognitive or emotional functioning; insufficient finances
Defining characteristics:
Objective: overtaxed family members (e.g., exhausted, anxious); unwashed or unavailable cooking equipment, clothes, or linen; repeated hygienic disorders, infestations, or infections; accumulation of dirt, food wastes, or hygienic wastes; disorderly surroundings; presence of vermin or rodents; inappropriate household temperature; lack of necessary equipment or aids; offensive odors
Subjective: household members express difficulty in maintaining their home in a comfortable fashion; household members describe outstanding debts or financial crises; household requests assistance with home maintenance

Hopelessness
Definition: subjective state in which an individual sees limited or no alternatives or personal choices available and is unable to mobilize energy on own behalf
Related factors: abandonment; prolonged activity restriction creating isolation; lost belief in transcendent values/God; long-term stress; failing or deteriorating physical condition
Defining characteristics: passivity; decreased verbalization; verbal cues (e.g., despondent content, "I can't," sighing); closing eyes; decreased affect; decreased appetite; decreased response to stimuli; increased/decreased sleep; lack of initiative; lack of involvement in care/passively allowing care; shrugging in response to speaker; turning away from speaker

Hyperthermia
Definition: body temperature elevated above normal range
Related factors: illness or trauma; increased metabolic rate; vigorous activity; medications or anesthesia; inability or decreased ability to perspire; (prolonged) exposure to hot environment; dehydration; inappropriate clothing
Defining characteristics: increase in body temperature above normal range; seizures or convulsions; flushed skin; increased respiratory rate; tachycardia; (skin) warm to touch

Hypothermia
Definition: body temperature below normal range
Related factors: exposure to cool or cold environment; medications causing vasodilation; malnutrition; inadequate clothing; illness or trauma; evaporation from skin in cool environment; decreased metabolic rate; damage to hypothalamus; consumption of alcohol; aging; inability or decreased ability to shiver; inactivity
Defining characteristics: pallor; reduction in body temperature below normal range; shivering; cool skin; cyanotic nail beds; hypertension; piloerection; slow capillary refill; tachycardia

Identity, disturbed personal
Definition: inability to distinguish between self and nonself
Related factors: to be developed
Defining characteristics: to be developed

Incontinence, bowel
Definition: change in normal bowel habits characterized by involuntary passage of stool
Related factors: environmental factors (e.g., inaccessible bathroom); incomplete emptying of bowel; rectal sphincter abnormality; impaction; dietary habits; colorectal lesions; stress; lower motor nerve damage; abnormally high abdominal or intestinal pressure; general decline in muscle tone; loss of rectal sphincter control; impaired cognition; upper motor nerve damage; chronic diarrhea; self-care deficit-toileting; impaired reservoir capacity; medications; immobility; laxative abuse
Defining characteristics: constant dribbling of soft stool; fecal odor; inability to delay defecation; urgency; self-report of inability to feel rectal fullness; fecal staining of clothing and/or bedding; recognizes rectal fullness but reports inability to expel formed stool; inattention to urge to defecate; inability to recognize urge to defecate; red perianal skin

Incontinence, functional urinary
Definition: inability of usually continent person to reach toilet in time to avoid unintentional loss of urine
Related factors: psychological factors; impaired vision; impaired cognition; neuromuscular limitations; altered environmental factors; weakened supporting pelvic structures
Defining characteristics: may only be incontinent in early morning; senses need to void; amount of time required to reach toilet exceeds length of time between sensing urge and uncontrolled voiding; loss of urine before reaching toilet; able to completely empty bladder

Incontinence, reflex urinary
Definition: involuntary loss of urine at somewhat predictable intervals when a specific bladder volume is reached
Related factors: tissue damage from radiation cystitis, inflammatory bladder conditions, or radical pelvic surgery; neurological impairment above level of sacral micturition center or pontine micturition center
Defining characteristics: no sensation of urge to void; complete emptying with lesion above pontine micturition center; incomplete emptying with lesion above sacral micturition center; no sensation of bladder fullness; sensations associated with full bladder such as sweating, restlessness, and abdominal discomfort; unable to cognitively inhibit or initiate voiding; no sensation of voiding; predictable pattern of voiding; sensation to urinate without voluntary inhibition of bladder contraction

Incontinence, stress urinary
Definition: less than 50 ml of urine occurring with increased abdominal pressure
Related factors: weak pelvic muscles and structural supports; over distention between voidings; incompetent bladder outlet; degenerative changes in pelvic muscles and structural supports associated with increased age; high intra-abdominal pressure (e.g., obesity, gravid uterus)
Defining characteristics: reported or observed dribbling with increased abdominal pressure; urinary frequency (more often than every two hours); urinary urgency

Incontinence, total urinary
Definition: continuous and unpredictable loss of urine
Related factors: neuropathy preventing transmission of reflex indicating bladder fullness; trauma or disease affecting spinal cord nerves; anatomic (fistula); independent contraction of detrusor reflex due to surgery; neurological dysfunction causing triggering of micturition at unpredictable times
Defining characteristics: constant flow of urine occurs at unpredictable times without distention or uninhibited bladder contractions/spasm; nocturia; unsuccessful incontinence refractory treatments; unawareness of incontinence; lack of perineal or bladder filling awareness

Incontinence, urge urinary
Definition: involuntary passage of urine occurring soon after a strong sense of urgency to void
Related factors: alcohol; caffeine; decreased bladder capacity (e.g., history of pelvic inflammatory disease [PID], abdominal surgeries, indwelling urinary catheter); increased fluid intake; increased urine concentration; irritation of bladder stretch receptors causing spasm (e.g., bladder infection); over distention of bladder
Defining characteristics: urinary urgency; bladder contracture/spasm; frequency (voiding more often than every two hours); voiding in large amounts (more than 550 cc); voiding in small amounts (less than 100 cc); nocturia (more than two times a night); inability to reach toilet in time

Incontinence, risk for urge urinary
Definition: at risk for involuntary loss of urine associated with a sudden, strong sensation or urinary urgency
Risk factors: effects of medications, caffeine, alcohol; detrusor hyperreflexia from cystitis, urethritis, tumors, renal calculi, central nervous system disorders above pontine micturition center; detrusor

muscle instability with impaired contractility; involuntary sphincter relaxation; ineffective toileting habits; small bladder capacity

Infant behavior, disorganized
Definition: disintegrated physiological and neurobehavioral responses to the environment
Related factors:
Prenatal: congenital or genetic disorders; teratogenic exposure
Postnatal: malnutrition; oral/motor problems; pain; feeding intolerance; invasive/painful procedures; prematurity
Individual: illness; immature neurological system; gestational age; postconceptual age
Environmental: physical environment inappropriateness; sensory inappropriateness; sensory overstimulation; sensory deprivation
Caregiver: cue misreading; cue knowledge deficit; environmental stimulation contribution
Defining characteristics:
Regulatory problems: inability to inhibit (inability to look away from stimulus); irritability
State-organization system: active-awake (fussy, worried gaze); diffuse/unclear sleep; state oscillation; quiet-awake (staring, gaze aversion); irritable or panicky crying
Attention-interaction system: abnormal response to sensory stimuli (e.g., difficult to soothe, inability to sustain alert status)
Motor system: increased, decreased, or limp tone; finger splay, fisting or hands to face; hyperextension of arms and legs; tremors, startles, twitches, jittery, jerky, uncoordinated movement; altered primitive reflexes
Physiological: bradycardia, tachycardia, or arrhythmias; pale, cyanotic, mottled, or flushed color; bradypnea, tachypnea, apnea; "time-out signals" (e.g., gaze, grasp, hiccup, cough, sneeze, sigh, slack jaw, open mouth, tongue thrust); oximeter desaturation; feeding intolerance (aspiration or emesis)

Infant behavior, risk for disorganized
Definition: risk for alteration in integrating and modulation of physiological and behavioral systems of functioning (i.e., autonomic, motor, state, organizational, self-regulatory, and attentional-interactional systems)
Risk factors: invasive/painful procedures; lack of containment/boundaries; oral/motor problems; pain; prematurity; environmental overstimulation

Infant behavior, readiness for enhanced organized
Definition: a pattern of modulation of the physiologic and behavioral systems of functioning (i.e., autonomic, motor, state organizational, self-regulators, and attentional-interactional systems) in an infant that is satisfactory but that can be improved, resulting in higher levels of integration in response to environmental stimuli
Related factors: pain; prematurity
Defining characteristics: definite sleep-wake states; use of some self-regulatory behaviors; response to visual/auditory stimuli; stable physiologic measures

Infant feeding pattern, ineffective
Definition: impaired ability to suck or coordinate the suck-swallow response
Related factors: prolonged NPO; anatomic abnormality; neurological impairment/delay; oral hyper-sensitivity; prematurity
Defining characteristics: inability to coordinate sucking, swallowing and breathing; inability to initiate or sustain an effective suck

Infection, risk for
Definition: at increased risk for being invaded by pathogenic organisms
Risk factors: invasive procedures; insufficient knowledge to avoid exposure to pathogens; trauma; tissue destruction and increased environmental exposure; rupture of amniotic membranes; pharmaceutical agents; malnutrition; increased environmental exposure; immunosuppression; inadequate acquired immunity; inadequate secondary defenses (decreased hemoglobin, leukopenia, suppressed inflammatory response); inadequate primary defenses (broken skin, traumatized tissue, decrease in ciliary action, stasis of body fluids, change in pH secretions, altered peristalsis); chronic disease

Injury, risk for
Definition: at risk of injury as a result of environmental conditions interacting with the individual's adaptive and defensive resources
Risk factors:
External: mode of transport or transportation; people or provider (e.g., nosocomial agents, staffing patterns, cognitive, affective and psychomotor factors); physical (e.g., design, structure, and arrangement of community, building and/or equipment); nutrients (e.g., vitamins, food types); biological (e.g., immunization level of community, microorganism); chemical (e.g., pollutants, poisons, drugs, pharmaceutical agents, alcohol, caffeine, nicotine, preservatives, cosmetics, and dyes)
Internal: psychological (affective orientation); malnutrition; abnormal blood profile (e.g., leukocytosis/leukopenia); altered clotting factors; thrombocytopenia; sickle cell; thalassemia; decreased hemoglobin; immune-autoimmune dysfunction; biochemical, regulatory function (e.g., sensory dysfunction); integrative dysfunction; effector dysfunction; tissue hypoxia; developmental age (physiological, psychosocial); physical (e.g., broken skin, altered mobility)

Injury, risk for perioperative positioning
Definition: at risk for injury as a result of the environmental conditions found in the perioperative setting
Risk factors: disorientation; edema; emaciation; immobilization, muscle weakness; obesity; sensory/perceptual disturbances due to anesthesia

Knowledge deficit (specify)
Definition: absence or deficiency of cognitive information related to a specific topic
Related factors: cognitive limitation; information misinterpretation; lack of exposure; lack of interest in learning; lack of recall; unfamiliarity with information resources
Defining characteristics: verbalization of the problem; inappropriate or exaggerated behaviors (e.g., hysterical, hostile, agitated, apathetic); inaccurate follow-through of instruction; inaccurate performance of test

Knowledge (specify), readiness for enhanced

Definition: the presence or acquisition of cognitive information related to a specific topic is sufficient for meeting health-related goals and can be strengthened

Defining characteristics: expresses an interest in learning; explains knowledge of the topic; behaviors congruent with expressed knowledge; describes previous experiences pertaining to the topic

Loneliness, risk for

Definition: at risk of experiencing vague dysphoria

Risk factors: affectional deprivation; social isolation; cathetic deprivation; physical isolation

Memory, impaired

Definition: inability to remember or recall bits of information or behavioral skills; may be attributed to pathophysiological or situational causes that are either temporary or permanent

Related factors: fluid and electrolyte imbalance; neurological disturbances; excessive environmental disturbances; anemia; acute or chronic hypoxia; decreased cardiac output

Defining characteristics: inability to recall factual information; inability to recall recent or past events; inability to learn or retain new skills or information; inability to determine if a behavior was performed; observed or reported experiences of forgetting; inability to perform a previously learned skill; forgets to perform a behavior at a scheduled time

Mobility, impaired bed

Definition: limitation of independent movement from one bed position to another (specify level)

Suggested Functional Level Classification:

0 = is completely independent

1 = requires use of equipment or device

2 = requires help from another person for assistance, supervision, or teaching

3 = requires help from another person and equipment/device

4 = is dependent; does not participate in activity

Related factors: to be developed

Defining characteristics: impaired ability to turn side to side; impaired ability to move from supine to sitting or sitting to supine; impaired ability to "scoot" or reposition self in bed; impaired ability to move from supine to prone or prone to supine; impaired ability to move from supine to long sitting or long sitting to supine

Mobility, impaired physical

Definition: limitation in independent, purposeful physical movement of the body or of one or more extremities (specify level)

Suggested Functional Level Classification:

0 = is completely independent

1 = requires use of equipment or device

2 = requires help from another person, for assistance, supervision, or teaching

3 = requires help from another person and equipment/device

4 = is dependent; does not participate in activity

Related factors: medications; prescribed movement restrictions; discomfort; lack of knowledge regarding value of physical activity; body mass index above 75th age-appropriate percentile; sensoriperceptual impairments; neuromuscular impairment; pain; musculoskeletal impairment; intolerance to activity/ decreased strength and endurance; depressive mood state or anxiety; cognitive impairment; decreased muscle strength, control and/or mass; reluctance to initiate movement; sedentary lifestyle or disuse or deconditioning; selective or generalized malnutrition; loss of integrity of bone structures; developmental delay; joint stiffness or contractures; limited cardiovascular endurance; altered cellular metabolism; lack of physical or social environmental supports; cultural beliefs regarding age appropriate activity

Defining characteristics: postural instability during performance of routine activities of daily living; limited ability to perform gross motor skills; limited ability to perform fine motor skills; uncoordinated or jerky movements; limited range of motion; difficulty turning; decreased reaction time; movement-induced shortness of breath; gait changes (e.g., decreased walk, speed, difficulty initiating gait, small steps, shuffles feet, exaggerated lateral postural sway); engages in substitutions for movement (e.g., increased attention to other's activity, controlling behavior, focus on pre-illness/disability activity); slowed movement; movement-induced tremor

Mobility, impaired wheelchair

Definition: limitation of independent operation of wheelchair within environment (specify level)

Suggested Functional Level Classification:

0 = is completely independent

1 = requires use of equipment or device

2 = requires help from another person for assistance, supervision, or teaching

3 = requires help from another person and equipment/device

4 = is dependent; does not participate in activity

Related factors: to be developed

Defining characteristics: impaired ability to operate manual or power wheelchair on even or uneven surface; impaired ability to operate manual or power wheelchair on an incline or decline; impaired ability to operate wheelchair on curbs

Nausea

Definition: a subjective unpleasant, wave-like sensation in the back of the throat, epigastrium, or throughout the abdomen that may or may not lead to vomiting

Related factors

Treatment related: gastric irritation (pharmaceuticals [e.g., aspirin, nonsteroidal anti-inflammatory drugs, steroids, antibiotics, alcohol, iron, and blood]); gastric distention (delayed gastric emptying caused by pharmacological interventions [e.g., narcotics administration, anesthesia agents]); pharmaceuticals (e.g., analgesics, antiviral for HIV, aspirin, opioids, chemotherapeutic agents); toxins (e.g., radio-therapy)

Biophysical: biochemical disorders (e.g., uremia, diabetic ketoacidosis, pregnancy); cardiac pain; cancer of stomach or intra-abdominal tumors (e.g., pelvic or colorectal cancers); esophageal or pancreatic disease; gastric distention due to delayed gastric emptying, pyloric intestinal obstruction, genitourinary and biliary distension, upper bowel stasis, external compression of the stomach, liver, spleen, or other organ enlargement that slows the stomach functioning (squashed stomach syndrome), excess food intake; gastric irritation due to pharyngeal and/or peritoneal inflammation; liver or splenic capsule stretch; local

tumors (e.g., acoustic neuroma, primary or secondary brain tumors, bone metastases at base of skull); motion sickness, Meniere's disease, or labyrinthitis; physical factors (e.g., increased intracranial pressure, meningitis); toxins (e.g., tumor-produced peptides, abnormal metabolites due to cancer)
Situational: psychological factors (e.g., pain, fear, anxiety, noxious odors, taste, unpleasant visual stimulation)
Defining characteristics: report of nausea ("sick to my stomach"); increased salivation; aversion toward food; gagging sensation; sour taste in mouth; increased swallowing

Neglect, unilateral
Definition: lack of awareness and attention to one side of the body
Related factors: effects of disturbed perceptual abilities (e.g., hemianopsia); neurologic illness or trauma; one-sided blindness
Defining characteristics: consistent inattention to stimuli on an affected side; does not look toward affected side; positioning and/or safety precautions in regard to the affected side; inadequate self-care; leaves food on plate on the affected side

Noncompliance (specify)
Definition: behavior of person and/or caregiver fails to coincide with a health-promoting or therapeutic plan agreed upon by the person (and/or family, and/or community) and health care professional. In the presence of an agreed-upon, health-promoting or therapeutic plan, person's or caregiver's behavior may be fully, partially, or nonadherent and may lead to clinically effective, partially effective, or ineffective outcomes.
Related factors:
Health care plan: duration; significant others; cost; intensity; complexity
Individual factors: personal and developmental abilities; health beliefs; cultural influences; spiritual values; individual's value system; knowledge and skill relevant to the regime behavior; motivational forces
Health system: satisfaction with care; credibility of provider; access and convenience of care; financial flexibility of plan; client-provider relationships; provider reimbursement of teaching and follow-up; provider continuity and regular follow-up; individual health coverage; communication and teaching skills of the provider
Network: involvement of members in health plan; social value regarding plan; perceived beliefs of significant others
Defining characteristics: behavior indicative of failure to adhere (by direct observation or by statements of patient or significant others); evidence of development of complications; evidence of exacerbation of symptoms; failure to keep appointments; failure to progress; objective tests (e.g., physiological measures, detection of physiologic markers)

Nutrition, imbalanced: less than body requirements
Definition: intake of nutrients insufficient to meet metabolic needs
Related factors: inability to ingest or digest food or absorb nutrients due to biological, psychological, or economic factors
Defining characteristics: pale conjunctival and mucous membranes; weakness of muscles required for swallowing or mastication; sore, inflamed buccal cavity; satiety immediately after ingesting food;

reported or evidence of lack of food; reported inadequate food intake less than RDA (recommended daily allowance); reported altered taste sensation; perceived inability to ingest food; misconceptions; loss of weight with adequate food intake; aversion to eating; abdominal cramping; poor muscle tone; abdominal pain with or without pathology; lack of interest in food; body weight 20% or more under ideal; capillary fragility; diarrhea and/or steatorrhea; excessive loss of hair; hyperactive bowel sounds; lack of information, misinformation

Nutrition, imbalanced: more than body requirements
Definition: intake of nutrients that exceeds metabolic needs
Related factors: excessive intake in relation to metabolic need
Defining characteristics: triceps skin fold greater than 25 mm in women; weight 20% over ideal for height and frame; triceps skin fold greater than 15 mm in men; eating in response to external cues, such as time of day, social situation; eating in response to internal cues other than hunger (e.g., anxiety); reported or observed dysfunctional eating pattern pairing food with other activities; sedentary activity level; concentrating food intake at the end of the day

Nutrition, imbalanced: risk for more than body requirements
Definition: at risk of experiencing an intake of nutrients that exceeds metabolic needs
Risk factors: reported use of solid food as major food source before five months of age; concentrating food intake at end of day; reported or observed obesity in one or both parents; reported or observed higher baseline weight at beginning of each pregnancy; rapid transition across growth percentiles in infants or children; pairing food with other activities; observed use of food as reward or comfort measure; eating in response to internal cues other than hunger, such as anxiety; eating in response to external cues such as time of day, social situation; dysfunctional eating patterns

Nutrition, readiness for enhanced
Definition: a pattern of nutrient intake that is sufficient for meeting metabolic needs and can be strengthened
Defining characteristics: expresses willingness to enhance nutrition; eats regularly; consumes adequate food and fluid; expresses knowledge of health food and fluid choices; follows an appropriate standard for intake (e.g., the food pyramid or America[n] Diabetic Association guidelines); safe preparation and storage for food and fluids; attitude toward eating and drinking is congruent with health goals

Oral mucous membrane, impaired
Definition: disruption of the lips and soft tissue of the oral cavity
Related factors: chemotherapy; chemical (e.g., alcohol, tobacco, acidic foods, regular use of inhalers); depression; immunosuppression; aging-related loss of connective, adipose, or bone tissue; barriers to professional care; cleft lip or palate; medication side effects; lack of or decreased salivation; trauma (chemical, e.g., acidic foods, drugs, noxious agents, alcohol); pathological conditions—oral cavity (radiation to head or neck); NPO for more than 24 hours; mouth breathing; malnutrition or vitamin deficiency; dehydration; infection; ineffective oral hygiene; mechanical (e.g., ill-fitting dentures, braces, tubes [endotracheal/nasogastric], surgery in oral cavity); decreased platelets; immunocompromised; impaired salivation; radiation therapy; barriers to oral self-care; diminished hormone levels (women); stress; loss of supportive structures

Defining characteristics: purulent drainage or exudates; gingival recession, pockets deeper than 4 mm; enlarged tonsils beyond what is developmentally appropriate; smooth atrophic, sensitive tongue; geographic tongue; mucosal dendation; presence of pathogens; difficult speech; self-report of bad taste; gingival or mucosal pallor; oral pain/discomfort; xerostomia (dry mouth); vesicles, nodules, or papules; white patches/plaques, spongy patches or white curd-like exudate; oral lesions or ulcers; halitosis; edema; hyperemia; desquamation; coated tongue; stomatitis; self-report of difficulty eating or swallowing; self-report of diminished or absent taste; bleeding; macroplasia; gingival hyperplasia; fissures, chelitis; red or bluish masses (e.g., hemangiomas)

Pain, acute
Definition: unpleasant sensory and emotional experience arising from actual or potential tissue damage or described in terms of such damage (International Association for the Study of Pain); sudden or slow onset of any intensity from mild to severe and a duration of less than six months
Related factors: injuring agents (biological, chemical, physical, psychological)
Defining characteristics: verbal or coded report; observed evidence (of pain); antalgic position; protective behavior; guarding behavior; antalgic gestures; facial mask; sleep disturbance (eyes lackluster, "hecohe [beaten] look," fixed or scattered movement, grimace); self-focus; narrowed focus (altered time perception, impaired thought processes, reduced interaction with people and environment); distraction behavior (e.g., pacing, seeking out other people and/or activities, repetitive activities); autonomic responses (e.g., diaphoresis, blood pressure, respiration, pulse change, pupillary dilation); autonomic alteration in muscle tone (may span from listless to rigid); expressive behavior (e.g., restlessness, moaning, crying, vigilance, irritability, sighing); changes in appetite and eating

Pain, chronic
Definition: unpleasant sensory and emotional experience arising from actual or potential tissue damage or described in terms of such damage (International Association for the Study of Pain); sudden or slow onset of any intensity from mild to severe, constant or recurring without an anticipated or predictable end and a duration of greater than 6 months
Related factors: chronic physical/psychosocial disability (e.g., cancer, arthritis)
Defining characteristics: weight changes; verbal or coded report or observed evidence of protective behavior; verbal or coded report or observed evidence of guarding behavior; verbal or coded report or observed evidence of facial mask; verbal or coded report or observed evidence of irritability; verbal or coded report or observed evidence of self-focusing; verbal or coded report or observed evidence of restlessness; verbal or coded report or observed evidence of depression; atrophy of involved muscle group; changes in sleep pattern; fatigue; fear of reinjury; reduced interaction with people; altered ability to continue previous activities; sympathetic mediated responses (e.g., temperature, cold, changes of body position, hypersensitivity); anorexia

Parenting, readiness for enhanced
Definition: a pattern of providing an environment for children or other dependent person(s) that is sufficient to nurture growth and development and can be strengthened
Defining characteristics: expresses willingness to enhance parenting; children or other dependent person(s) express satisfaction with home environment; emotional and tacit support of children or

dependent person(s) is evident; bonding or attachment evident; physical and emotional needs of children/dependent person(s) are met; realistic expectations of children/dependent person(s) exhibited

Parenting, impaired
Definition: inability of the primary caretaker to create an environment that promotes the optimum growth and development of the child
Related factors:
Social: lack of access to resources; social isolation; lack of resources; poor home environments; lack of family cohesiveness; inadequate child care arrangements; lack of transportation; unemployment or job problems; role strain or overload; marital conflict, declining satisfaction; lack of value of parenthood; change in family unit; low socioeconomic class; unplanned or unwanted pregnancy; presence of stress (e.g., financial, legal, recent crisis, cultural move); lack of, or poor, parental role model; single parents; lack of social support networks; father or child not involved; history of being abusive; history of being abused; financial difficulties; maladaptive coping strategies; poverty; poor problem-solving skills; inability to put child's needs before own; low self-esteem; relocations; legal difficulties
Knowledge: lack of knowledge about child health maintenance; lack of knowledge about parenting skills; unrealistic expectation for self, infant, partner; limited cognitive functioning; lack of knowledge about child development; inability to recognize and act on infant cues; low educational level or attainment; poor communication skills; lack of cognitive readiness for parenthood; preference for physical punishment
Physiological: physical illness
Infant or child: premature birth; illness; prolonged separation from parent; not gender desired; attention deficit hyperactivity disorder; difficult temperament; separation from parent at birth; lack of goodness of fit (temperament) with parental expectations; unplanned or unwanted child; handicapping condition or developmental delay; multiple births; altered perceptual abilities
Psychological: history of substance abuse or dependencies; disability; depression; difficult labor and/or delivery; young age, especially adolescent; history of mental illness; high number of closely spaced pregnancies; sleep deprivation or disruption; lack of, or late, prenatal care; separation from infant/child; multiple births
Defining characteristics:
Infant or child: poor academic performance; frequent illness; runaway; incidence of physical and psychological trauma or abuse; frequent accidents; lack of attachment; failure to thrive; behavioral disorders; poor social competence; lack of separation anxiety; poor cognitive development
Parental: inappropriate child care arrangements; rejection or hostility to child; statement of inability to meet child's needs; inflexibility to meet needs of child, situation; poor or inappropriate catering skills; high punitiveness; inconsistent care; child abuse; inadequate child health maintenance; unsafe home environment; verbalization, cannot control child; negative statements about child; verbalization of role inadequacy frustration; inappropriate visual, tactile, auditory stimulation; inappropriate child care arrangements; abandonment; insecure or lack of attachment to infant; inconsistent behavior management; child neglect; little cuddling; maternal-child interaction deficit; poor parent-child interaction

Parenting, risk for impaired
Definition: risk for inability of the primary caretaker to create, maintain, or regain an environment that promotes the optimum growth and development of the child

Risk factors:

Social: marital conflict, declining satisfaction; history of being abused; poor problem solving skills; role strain/overload; social isolation; legal difficulties; lack of access to resources; lack of value of parenthood; relocation; poverty; poor home environment; lack of family cohesiveness; lack of poor parental role model; father of child not involved; history of being abused; financial difficulties; low self-esteem; unplanned or unwanted pregnancy; inadequate child care arrangements; maladaptive coping strategies; lack of resources; low socioeconomic class; lack of transportation; change in family unit; unemployment or job problems; single parent; lack of social support network; inability to put child's needs before own; stress

Knowledge: low educational level or attainment; unrealistic expectations of child; lack of knowledge about parenting skills; poor communication skills; preference for physical punishment; inability to recognize and act on infant cues; low cognitive functioning; lack of knowledge about child health maintenance; lack of knowledge about child development; lack of cognitive readiness for parenthood

Physiological: physical illness

Infant or child: multiple births; handicapping condition or developmental delay; illness; altered perceptual abilities; lack of goodness of fit (temperament) with parental expectations; unplanned or unwanted child; premature birth; not gender desired; difficult temperament; attention deficit hyperactivity disorder; prolonged separation from parent; separation from parent at birth

Psychological: separation from infant/child; high number of closely spaced children; disability; sleep deprivation or disruption; multiple births; difficult labor and/or delivery; young ages, especially adolescent; depression; history of mental illness; lack of, or late, prenatal care; history of substance abuse or dependence

Peripheral neurovascular dysfunction, risk for

Definition: at risk of experiencing a disruption in circulation, sensation or motion of an extremity

Risk factors: trauma; vascular obstruction; orthopedic surgery; fractures; burns; mechanical compression (e.g., tourniquet, cast, brace, dressing or restraint); immobilization

Poisoning, risk for

Definition: accentuated risk of accidental exposure to or ingestion of drugs or dangerous products in doses sufficient to cause poisoning

Risk factors:

External: unprotected contact with heavy metals or chemicals; medicines stored in unlocked cabinets accessible to children or confused people; presence of poisonous vegetation; presence of atmospheric pollutants; paint, lacquer, etc., in poorly ventilated areas or without effective protection; flaking, peeling paint or plaster in presence of young children; chemical contamination of food and water; availability of illicit drugs potentially contaminated by poisonous additives; large supplies of drugs in house; dangerous products placed or stored within reach of children or confused people

Internal: verbalization of occupational setting without adequate safeguards; reduced vision; lack of safety or drug education; lack of proper precaution; insufficient finances; cognitive or emotional difficulties

Post-trauma syndrome

Definition: sustained maladaptive response to a traumatic, overwhelming event

Related factors: events outside the range of usual human experience; physical and psychosocial abuse; tragic occurrence involving multiple deaths; sudden destruction of one's home or community; epidemics;

being held prisoner of war or criminal victimization (torture); wars; rape; natural disasters and/or man-made disasters; serious accidents; witnessing mutilation, violent death, or other horrors; serious threat or injury to self or loved ones; industrial and motor vehicle accidents; military combat

Defining characteristics: avoidance; repression; difficulty in concentrating; grief; intrusive thoughts; neurosensory irritability; palpitations; enuresis (in children); anger and/or rage; intrusive dreams; nightmares; aggression; hypervigilant; exaggerated startle response; hopelessness; altered mood states; shame; panic attacks; alienation; denial; horror; substance abuse; depression; anxiety; guilt; fear; gastric irritability; detachment; psychogenic amnesia; irritability; numbing; compulsive behavior; flashbacks; headaches

Post-trauma syndrome, risk for

Definition: at risk for sustained maladaptive response to a traumatic, overwhelming event

Risk factors: occupation (e.g., police, fire, rescue, corrections, emergency room staff, mental health); exaggerated sense of responsibility; perception of event; survivor's role in the event; displacement from home; inadequate social support; non-supportive environment; diminished ego strength; duration of the event

Powerlessness

Definition: perception that one's own action will not significantly affect an outcome; a perceived lack of control over a current situation or immediate happening

Related factors: health care environment; illness-related regime; interpersonal interaction; lifestyle of helplessness

Defining characteristics:

Low: expressions of uncertainty about fluctuating energy levels; passivity

Moderate: nonparticipation in care or decision making when opportunities are provided; resentment; anger; guilt; reluctance to express true feelings; passivity; dependence on others that may result in irritability; fearing alienation from caregivers; expressions of dissatisfaction and frustration over inability to perform previous tasks and/or activities; expression of doubt regarding role performance; does not monitor progress; does not defend self-care practices when challenged; inability to seek information regarding care

Severe: verbal expressions of having no control or influence over self-care, situation, or outcome; apathy; depression over physical deterioration that occurs despite patient compliance with regimens

Powerlessness, risk for

Definition: at risk for perceived lack of control over a situation and/or one's ability to significantly affect an outcome

Risk factors:

Physiological: chronic or acute illness (hospitalization, intubation, ventilator, suctioning); acute injury or progressive debilitating disease process (e.g., spinal cord injury, multiple sclerosis); aging (e.g., decreased physical strength, decreased mobility); dying

Psychosocial: lack of knowledge of illness or healthcare system; lifestyle of dependency with inadequate coping patterns; absence of integrality (e.g., essence of power); decreased self esteem; low or unstable body image

Protection, ineffective

Definition: decrease in the ability to guard self from internal or external threat such as illness or injury

Related factors: abnormal blood profiles (e.g., leukopenia, thrombocytopenia, anemia, coagulation); inadequate nutrition; extremes of age; drug therapies (e.g., antineoplastic, corticosteroid, immune, anticoagulant, thrombolytic); alcohol abuse; treatments (e.g., surgery, radiation); diseases such as cancer and immune disorders

Defining characteristics: maladaptive stress response; neuro-sensory alteration; impaired healing; deficient immunity; altered clotting; dyspnea; insomnia; weakness; restlessness; pressure ulcers; perspiring; itching; immobility; fatigue; anorexia

Rape-trauma syndrome

Definition: sustained maladaptive response to a forced, violent sexual penetration against the victim's will and consent

Related factors: rape

Defining characteristics: disorganization; change in relationships; confusion; physical trauma (e.g., bruising, tissue irritation); suicide attempts; denial; guilt; paranoia; humiliation; embarrassment; aggression; muscle tension and/or spasms; mood swings; dependence; powerlessness; nightmares and sleep disturbances; sexual dysfunction; revenge; phobias; loss of self-esteem; inability to make decisions; dissociative disorders; self-blame; hyperalertness; vulnerability; substance abuse; depression; helplessness; anger; anxiety; agitation; shame; shock; fear

Note: this syndrome includes the following three sub-components: rape-trauma, compound reaction, and silent reaction. In this text each appears as a separate diagnosis.

Rape-trauma syndrome: compound reaction

Definition: forced violent sexual penetration against the victim's will and consent. The trauma syndrome that develops from this attack or attempted attack includes an acute phase of disorganization of the victim's lifestyle and a long-term process of reorganization of lifestyle.

Related factors: to be developed

Defining characteristics: change in lifestyle (e.g., changes in residence, dealing with repetitive nightmares and phobias, seeking family support, needing social network support in long-term phase); emotional reaction (e.g., anger, embarrassment, fear of physical violence and death, humiliation, revenge, self-blame in acute phase); multiple physical symptoms (e.g., gastrointestinal irritability, genitourinary discomfort, muscle tension, sleep pattern disturbance in acute phase); reactivated symptoms of such previous conditions (i.e., physical illness, psychiatric illness in acute phase); reliance on alcohol and/or drugs (acute phase)

Rape-trauma syndrome: silent reaction

Definition: forced violent sexual penetration against the victim's will and consent. The trauma syndrome that develops from this attack or attempted attack includes an acute phase of disorganization of the victim's lifestyle and a long-term process or reorganization of lifestyle.

Related factors: to be developed

Defining characteristics: increased anxiety during interview (i.e., blocking of associations, long periods of silence, minor stuttering, physical distress); sudden onset of phobic reaction; no verbalization of the occurrence of rape; abrupt changes in relationships with men; increase in nightmares; pronounced changes in sexual behavior

Religiosity, impaired
Definition: impaired ability to exercise reliance on beliefs and/or participate in rituals of a particular faith tradition
Related factors:
Physical: sickness/illness; pain
Psychological: ineffective support/coping; personal disaster/crisis; lack of security; anxiety; fear of death; ineffective coping with disease; use of religion to manipulate
Sociocultural: barriers to practicing religion (cultural and environmental); lack of social integration; lack of social/cultural interaction
Spiritual: spiritual crises; suffering
Developmental and Situational: end stage life crises; life transitions; aging
Defining characteristics: demonstrates or explains difficulty adhering to prescribed **religious beliefs** and rituals, for example: religious ceremonies; dietary regulations; clothing; prayer; worship; religious services; private religious behaviors; reading religious materials; media; holiday observances; meetings with religious leaders; expresses emotional distress because of separation from faith community; expresses emotional distress regarding religious beliefs and/or religious social network; expresses a need to reconnect with previous belief patterns and customs; questions religious belief patterns and customs

Religiosity, risk for impaired
Definition: at risk for an impaired ability to exercise reliance on religious beliefs and/or participate in rituals of a particular faith tradition
Risk factors:
Physical: illness/hospitalization; pain
Psychological: ineffective support/coping/caregiving; depression; lack of security
Sociocultural: lack of social interaction; cultural barrier to practicing religion; social isolation
Spiritual: suffering
Environmental: lack of transportation; environmental barriers to practicing religion
Developmental: life transitions

Religiosity, readiness for enhanced
Definition: ability to increase reliance on religious beliefs and/or participate in rituals of a particular faith tradition
Defining characteristics: expresses desire to strengthen religious belief patterns and customs that had provided comfort/religion in the past; request for assistance to increase participation in prescribed religious beliefs through: religious ceremonies; dietary regulations/rituals; clothing; prayer; worship/ religious services; private religious behaviors/reading religious materials/media; holiday observances Requests assistance expanding religious options; requests meeting with religious leaders/facilitators; requests forgiveness, reconciliation; requests religious material and/or experiences; questions or rejects belief patterns and customs that are harmful

Relocation stress syndrome

Definition: physiological and/or psychosocial disturbances as a result of transfer from one environment to another

Related factors: impaired psychosocial health status; past, concurrent, and recent losses; moderate to high degree of environment change; losses involved with decision to move; lack of adequate support system; history and types of previous transfers; feeling of powerlessness; decreased physical health status; little or no preparation for the impending move

Defining characteristics: increased confusion; loneliness; depression; apprehension; anxiety; change in environment/location; sleep disturbance; withdrawal; weight change; vigilance; verbalization of unwillingness to relocate; verbalization of being concerned/upset about transfer; sad affect; restlessness; lack of trust; insecurity; increased verbalization of needs; gastrointestinal disturbances; dependency; change in eating habits; unfavorable comparison of post/pre-transfer staff

Relocation, stress syndrome risk for

Definition: at risk for physiological and/or psychosocial disturbance following transfer from one environment to another

Risk factors: moderate to high degree of environmental change (e.g., physical, ethnic, cultural); temporary and/or permanent moves; voluntary/involuntary move; lack of adequate support system/group; feelings of powerlessness; moderate mental competence (e.g., alert enough to experience changes); unpredictability of experiences; decreased psychosocial or physical health status; lack of predeparture counseling; passive coping; past, current, recent losses

Role performance, ineffective

Definition: patterns of behavior and self-expression do not match the environmental context, norms, and expectations

Related factors:

Social: inadequate or inappropriate linkage with the health care system; job schedule demands; young age, developmental level; lack of rewards; poverty; family conflict; inadequate support system; inadequate role socialization (e.g., role model, expectations, responsibilities); low social economic status; stress and conflict; domestic violence; lack of resources

Knowledge: inadequate role preparation (e.g., role transition, skill, rehearsal, validation); lack of knowledge about role; role transition; lack of opportunity for role rehearsal; developmental transitions; unrealistic role expectations; education attainment level; lack of or inadequate role model; lack of knowledge about role skills

Physiological: inadequate/inappropriate linkage with health care system; substance abuse; mental illness; body image alteration; physical illness; cognitive deficits; health alterations (e.g., physical health, body image, self-esteem, mental health, psychosocial health, cognition, learning style, neurological health); depression; low self-esteem; pain; fatigue

Defining characteristics: change in self-perception of role; role denial; inadequate external support for role enactment; inadequate adaptation to change or transition; system conflict; change in usual patterns of responsibility; discrimination; domestic violence; harassment; uncertainty; altered role perceptions; role strain; inadequate self-management; role ambivalence; pessimistic; inadequate motivation; inadequate confidence; inadequate role competency and skills; inadequate knowledge; inappropriate developmental expectations; role conflict; role confusion; powerlessness; inadequate coping; anxiety or depression; role overload; change in other's perception of role; change in capacity to resume role; role dissatisfaction; inadequate opportunities for role enactment

Sedentary life style
Definition: reports a habit of life that is characterized by a low physical activity level
Defining characteristics: chooses a daily routine lacking physical exercise; demonstrates physical deconditioning; verbalizes preference for activities low in physical activity
Related factors: deficient knowledge of health benefits of physical exercise; lack of motivation; lack of interest; lack of training for accomplishment of physical exercise; lack of resources: time, money, companionship, facilities

Self-care deficit, bathing/hygiene
Definition: impaired ability to perform or complete bathing/hygiene activities for oneself (see Suggested Functional Level Classification under diagnosis *Impaired Physical Mobility*)
Risk factors: discomfort
Related factors: decreased or lack of motivation; weakness and tiredness; severe anxiety; inadequate to perceive body part or spatial relationship; perceptual or cognitive impairment; pain; neuromuscular impairment; musculoskeletal impairment; environmental barriers
Defining characteristics: inability to get bath supplies; inability to wash body or body parts; inability to obtain or get to water source; inability to regulate temperature or flow of bath water; inability to get in and out of bathroom; inability to dry body

Self-care deficit, dressing/grooming
Definition: impaired ability to perform or complete dressing and grooming activities for oneself (see Suggested Functional Level Classification under diagnosis *Impaired Physical Mobility*)
Related factors: decreased or lack of motivation; pain; severe anxiety; perceptual or cognitive impairment; neuromuscular impairment; musculoskeletal impairment; discomfort; environmental barriers; weakness or tiredness
Defining characteristics: inability to choose clothing; inability to use assistive devices; inability to use zippers; inability to remove clothes; inability to put on socks; inability to put on clothing on upper body; impaired ability to put on or take off necessary items of clothing; impaired ability to fasten clothing; impaired ability to obtain or replace articles of clothing; inability to maintain appearance at a satisfactory level; inability to put on clothing on lower body; inability to pick up clothing; inability to put on shoes

Self-care deficit, feeding
Definition: impaired ability to perform or complete feeding activities (see Suggested Functional Level Classification under *Impaired Physical Mobility*)
Related factors: weakness or tiredness; severe anxiety; neuromuscular impairment; pain; perceptual or cognitive impairment; discomfort; environmental barriers; decreased or lack of motivation; musculoskeletal impairments

Defining characteristics: inability to swallow food; inability to prepare food for ingestion; inability to handle utensils; inability to chew food; inability to use assistive device; inability to get food onto utensil; inability to open containers; inability to manipulate food in mouth; inability to ingest food safely; inability to bring food from a receptacle to the mouth; inability to complete a meal; inability to ingest food in a socially acceptable manner; inability to pick up cup or glass; inability to ingest sufficient food

Self-care deficit, toileting

Definition: impaired ability to perform or complete own toileting activities (see Suggested Functional Level Classification under *Impaired Physical Mobility*)

Related factors: environmental barriers; weakness or tiredness; decreased or lack of motivation; severe anxiety; impaired mobility status; impaired transfer ability; musculoskeletal impairment; neuromuscular impairment; pain; perceptual or cognitive impairment

Defining characteristics: inability to manipulate clothing, unable to carry out proper toilet hygiene; unable to sit on or rise from toilet or commode; unable to get to toilet or commode; unable to flush toilet or commode

Self-concept, readiness for enhanced

Definition: a pattern of perceptions or ideas about the self that is sufficient for well-being and can be strengthened

Defining characteristics: expresses willingness to enhance self-concept; expresses satisfaction with thoughts about self, sense of worthiness, role performance, body image, and personal identity; actions are congruent with expressed feelings and thoughts; expresses confidence in abilities; accepts strengths and limitations

Self-esteem, chronic low

Definition: long standing negative self-evaluation/feelings about self or self-capabilities

Related factors: to be developed

Defining characteristics: rationalizes away/rejects positive feedback and exaggerates negative feedback about self (long standing or chronic); self-negating verbalization (long standing or chronic); hesitant to try new things/situations (long standing or chronic); expressions of shame/guilt (long standing or chronic); evaluates self as unable to deal with events (long standing or chronic); lack of eye contact; nonassertive/passive; frequent lack of success in work or other life events; excessively seeks reassurance; overly conforming; dependent on others' opinions; indecisive

Self-esteem, situational low

Definition: negative self-evaluation/feelings about self that develop in response to a loss or change in an individual who previously had a positive self-evaluation

Related factors: to be developed

Defining characteristics: verbalization of negative feelings about self (e.g., helplessness, uselessness); episodic occurrence of negative self-appraisal in response to life events in a person with a previous positive self-evaluation; difficulty making decisions; evaluates self as unable to handle situations/events; expressions of shame/guilt; self-negating verbalizations

Self-esteem, risk for situational low

Definition: at risk for developing negative perception of self-worth in response to a current situation (specify)

Risk factors: developmental changes (specify); disturbed body image; functional impairment (specify); loss (specify); social role changes (specify); history of learned helplessness; history of abuse, neglect, or abandonment; unrealistic self-expectations; behavior inconsistent with values; lack of recognition/rewards; failures/rejections; decreased power/control over environment; physical illness (specify)

Self-mutilation

Definition: deliberate self-injurious behavior causing tissue damage with the intent of causing nonfatal injury to attain relief of tension

Related factors: psychotic state (command hallucinations); inability to express tension verbally; childhood sexual abuse; violence between parental figures; family divorce; family alcoholism; family history of self-destructive behaviors; adolescence; peers who self-mutilate; isolation from peers; perfectionism; substance abuse; eating disorders; sexual identity crisis; low or unstable self-esteem; low or unstable body image; labile behavior (mood swings); history of inability to plan solutions or see long-term consequences; use of manipulation to obtain nurturing relationship with others; chaotic/disturbed interpersonal relationships; emotionally disturbed; battered child; feels threatened with actual or potential loss of significant relationship (e.g., loss of parent/parental relationship); experiences dissociation or depersonalization; mounting tension that is intolerable; impulsivity; inadequate coping; irresistible urge to cut/damage self; needs quick reduction of stress; childhood illness or surgery; foster, group, or institutional care; incarceration; character disorder; borderline personality disorder; developmentally delayed or autistic individual; history of self-injurious behavior; feelings of depression, rejection, self-hatred, separation anxiety, guilt, depersonalization; poor parent-adolescent communication; lack of family confidant

Defining characteristics: cuts/scratches on body; picking at wounds; self-inflicted burns (e.g., eraser, cigarette); ingestion/inhalation of harmful substances/objects; biting; abrading; severing; insertion of object(s) into body orifice(s); hitting; constricting a body part

Self-mutilation, risk for

Definition: at high risk to perform an act upon the self to injure, not kill, which produces tissue damage and tension relief

Risk factors: command hallucinations; need for sensory stimuli; mentally retarded and autistic children; inability to cope with increased psychological/physiological tension in a healthy manner; history of physical, emotional, or sexual abuse; fluctuating emotions; feelings of depression, rejection, self-hatred, separation anxiety, guilt and depersonalization; dysfunctional family; clients with borderline personality disorder, especially females 16–25 years of age; clients with a history of self-injury; clients in psychotic state—frequently males in young adulthood; parental emotional deprivation; emotionally disturbed and/or battered children

Sensory/perceptual, disturbed (specify: auditory, gustatory, kinesthetic, olfactory, tactile, visual)

Definition: change in the amount or pattering of incoming stimuli accompanied by a diminished, exaggerated, distorted or impaired response to such stimuli

Related factors: altered sensory perception; excessive environmental stimuli; psychological stress; altered sensory reception, transmission, and/or integration; insufficient environmental stimuli; biochemical imbalances for sensory distortions (e.g., illusions, hallucinations); electrolyte imbalance; biochemical imbalance

Defining characteristics: poor concentration; auditory distortions; change in usual response to stimuli; restlessness; reported or measured change in sensory acuity; irritability; disoriented in time, in place, or with people; change in problem-solving abilities; change in behavior pattern; altered communication patterns; hallucinations; visual distortions

Sexual dysfunction

Definition: change in sexual function that is viewed as unsatisfying, unrewarding, inadequate
Related factors: misinformation or lack of knowledge; vulnerability; values conflict; psychosocial abuse (e.g., harmful relationships); physical abuse; lack of privacy; ineffectual or absent role models; altered body structure or function (e.g., pregnancy, recent childbirth, drugs, surgery, anomalies, disease process, trauma, radiation); lack of significant other; biopsychosocial alteration of sexuality
Defining characteristics: change of interest in self and others; conflicts involving values; inability to achieve desired satisfaction; verbalization of problem; alteration in relationship with significant other; alteration in achieving sexual satisfaction; actual or perceived limitations imposed by disease and/or therapy; seeking confirmation of desirability; alterations in achieving perceived sex role

Sexuality patterns, ineffective

Definition: expressions of concern regarding his/her sexuality
Related factors: lack of significant other; conflicts with sexual orientation or variant preferences; fear of pregnancy or of acquiring a sexually transmitted disease; impaired relationship with a significant other; ineffective or absent role models; knowledge/skill deficit about alternative responses to health-related transitions, altered body function or structure, illness or medical; lack of privacy
Defining characteristics: reported difficulties, limitations, or changes in sexual behaviors or activities

Skin integrity, impaired

Definition: altered epidermis and/or dermis
Related factors:
External: hyperthermia or hypothermia; chemical substance; humidity; mechanical factors (e.g., shearing forces, pressure, restraint); physical immobilization; radiation; extremes in age; moisture; altered fluid status; medications
Internal: altered metabolic state; skeletal prominence; immunological deficit; developmental factors; altered sensation; altered nutritional state (e.g., obesity, emaciation); altered pigmentation; altered circulation; alterations in turgor (changes in elasticity)
Defining characteristics: invasion of body structures; destruction of skin layers (dermis); disruption of skin surface (epidermis)

Skin integrity, risk for impaired

Definition: at risk of being adversely altered
Risk factors:
External: radiation; physical immobilization; mechanical factors (e.g., shearing forces, pressure, restraint); hypothermia or hyperthermia; humidity; chemical substance; excretions and/or secretions; moisture; extremes of age

Internal: medication; skeletal prominence; immunologic; developmental factors; altered sensation; altered pigmentation; altered metabolic state; altered circulation; alterations in skin turgor (changes in elasticity); alterations in nutritional state (e.g., obesity, emaciation); psychogenetic

Sleep deprivation
Definition: prolonged periods of time without sustained natural, periodic suspension of relative consciousness
Related factors: prolonged physical discomfort; prolonged psychological discomfort; sustained inadequate sleep hygiene; prolonged use of pharmacologic or dietary antisoporifics; aging-related sleep stage shifts; sustained circadian asynchrony; inadequate daytime activity; sustained environmental stimulation; sustained unfamiliar or uncomfortable sleep environment; nonsleep-inducing parenting practices; sleep apnea; periodic limb movement (e.g., restless leg syndrome, nocturnal myoclonus); sundowner's syndrome; narcolepsy; idiopathic central nervous system hypersomnolence; sleep walking; sleep terror; sleep-related enuresis; nightmares; familial sleep paralysis; sleep-related painful erections; dementia
Defining characteristics: daytime drowsiness; decreased ability to function; malaise; tiredness; lethargy; restlessness; irritability; heightened sensitivity to pain; listlessness; apathy; slowed reactional inability to concentrate; perceptual disorders (e.g., disturbed body sensation, delusions, feeling afloat); hallucinations; acute confusion; transient paranoia; agitated or combative; anxious; mild, fleeting nystagmus; hand tremors

Sleep pattern disturbed
Definition: time-limited disruption of sleep (natural, periodic suspension of consciousness) amount and quality
Related factors:
Psychological: ruminative pre-sleep thoughts; daytime activity pattern; thinking about home; body temperature; temperament; dietary; childhood onset; inadequate sleep hygiene; sustained use of anti-sleep agents; circadian asynchrony; frequently changing sleep-wake schedule; depression; loneliness; frequent travel across time zones; daylight/darkness exposure; grief; anticipation; shift work; delayed or advanced sleep phase syndrome; loss of sleep partner, life change; preoccupation with trying to sleep; periodic gender-related hormonal shifts; biochemical agents; fear; separation from significant others; social schedule inconsistent with chronotype; aging-related sleep shifts; anxiety; medications; fear of insomnia; maladaptive conditioned wakefulness; fatigue; boredom
Environmental: noise; unfamiliar sleep furnishings; ambient temperature; humidity; lighting; other-generated awakening; excessive stimulation; physical restraint; lack of sleep privacy/control; nurse for therapeutics, monitoring, lab tests; sleep partner; noxious odors
Parental: mother's sleep-wake pattern; parent-infant interaction; mother's emotional support
Physiological: urinary urgency; wet; fever, nausea; stasis of secretions; shortness of breath; position; gastroesophageal reflux
Defining characteristics: prolonged awakenings; sleep maintenance insomnia; self-induced impairment of normal pattern; sleep onset greater than 30 minutes; early morning insomnia; awakening earlier or later than desired; verbal complaints of difficulty falling asleep; verbal complaints of not feeling well-rested; increased proportion of stage 1 sleep; dissatisfaction with sleep; less than age-normed total

sleep time; three or more nighttime awakenings; decreased proportion of stages 3 and 4 sleep (e.g., hyporesponsiveness, excess sleepiness, decreased motivation); decreased proportion of REM sleep (e.g., rapid eye movement (REM) rebound, hyperactivity, emotional lability, agitation and impulsivity, atypical polysomnographic features); decreased ability to function

Sleep, readiness for enhanced
Definition: a pattern of natural, periodic suspension of consciousness that provides adequate rest, sustains a desired lifestyle, and can be strengthened
Defining characteristics: expresses willingness to enhance sleep; amount of sleep and REM sleep is congruent with developmental needs; expresses a feeling of being rested after sleep; follows sleep routines that promote sleep habits; occasional or infrequent use of medications to induce sleep

Social interaction, impaired
Definition: insufficient or excessive quantity or ineffective quality of social exchange
Related factors: knowledge/skill deficit about ways to enhance mutuality; therapeutic isolation; sociocultural dissonance; limited physical mobility; environmental barriers; communication barriers; altered thought processes; absence of available significant others or peers; self-concept disturbance
Defining characteristics: verbalized or observed inability to receive or communicate a satisfying sense of belonging, caring, interest, or shared history; verbalized or observed discomfort in social situations; observed use of unsuccessful social interaction behaviors; dysfunctional interaction with peers, family and/or others; family report of change of style or pattern of interaction

Social isolation
Definition: aloneness experienced by the individual and perceived as imposed by others and as a negative or threatening state
Related factors: alterations in mental status; inability to engage in satisfying personal relationships; unaccepted social values; unaccepted social behavior; inadequate personal resources; immature interests; factors contributing to the absence of satisfying personal relationships (e.g., delay in accomplishing developmental tasks); alterations in physical appearance; altered state of wellness
Defining characteristics:
Objective: absence of supportive significant other(s), family, friends, group; projects hostility in voice, behavior; withdrawn; uncommunicative; shows behavior unaccepted by dominant cultural group; seeks to be alone or exists in a subculture; repetitive, meaningless actions; preoccupation with own thoughts; no eye contact; evidence of physical/mental handicap or altered state of wellness; sad, dull affect
Subjective: expresses feeling of aloneness imposed by others; expresses feelings of rejection; inappropriate or immature interests/activities for development age/stage; inadequate or absent significant purpose in life; inability to meet expectation of others; expresses values acceptable to the subculture but unacceptable to the dominant cultural group; expresses interests inappropriate to the developmental age/stage; experiences feelings of differences from others; insecurity in public

Sorrow, chronic
Definition: cyclical, recurring and potentially progressive pattern of pervasive sadness that is experienced by a client (parent or caregiver, or individual with chronic illness or disability) in response to continual loss, throughout the trajectory of an illness or disability

Related factors: death of a loved one; person experiences chronic physical or mental illness or disability, such as mental retardation, multiple sclerosis, prematurity, spina bifida or other birth defects, infertility, cancer, Parkinson's disease; person experiences one or more trigger events (e.g., crises in management of the illness, crises related to developmental stages and missed opportunities or milestones that bring comparisons with developmental, social, or personal norms); unending caregiving as a constant reminder of loss

Defining characteristics: feelings that vary in intensity, are periodic, may progress and intensify over time, and may interfere with the client's ability to reach his/her highest level of personal and social well-being; client expresses periodic, recurrent feelings of sadness; client expresses one or more of the following feelings: anger, being misunderstood, confusion, depression, disappointment, emptiness, fear, frustration, guilt/self-blame, helplessness, hopelessness, loneliness, low self-esteem, recurring loss, overwhelmed

Spiritual distress

Definition: impaired ability to experience and integrate meaning and purpose in life through a person's connectedness with self, others, art, music, literature, nature, or a power greater than oneself

Related factors: self-alienation; loneliness/social alienation; anxiety; sociocultural deprivation; death and dying of self or others; pain; life change; chronic illness of self or others

Defining characteristics:

Connections to self: expresses lack of hope, meaning and purpose, peace/serenity, acceptance, love, forgiveness of self, courage; anger; guilt; poor coping

Connections with others: refuses interactions with spiritual leaders; refuses interaction with friends, family; verbalizes being separated from their support system; expresses alienation

Connections with art, music, literature, nature: inability to express previous state of creativity (singing/listening to music/writing); no interest in nature; no interest in reading spiritual literature

Connections with power greater than self: inability to pray; inability to participate in religious activities; expresses being abandoned by or having anger toward God; inability to experience the transcendent; requests to see a religious leader; sudden changes in spiritual practices; inability to be introspective/inward turning; expresses being without hope, suffering

Spiritual distress, risk for

Definition: at risk for an impaired ability to experience and integrate meaning and purpose in life through a person's connectedness with self, other persons, art, music, literature, nature, and/or a power greater than oneself

Risk factors:

Physical: physical illness; substance abuse/excessive drinking; chronic illness

Psychosocial: low self-esteem; depression; anxiety; stress; poor relationships; separate from support systems; blocks to experiencing love; inability to forgive; loss; racial/cultural conflict; change in religious rituals; change in spiritual practices

Developmental: life change; developmental life changes

Environmental: environmental changes; natural disasters

Spiritual well-being, readiness for enhanced

Definition: ability to experience and integrate meaning and purpose in life through connectedness with self, others, art, music, literature, nature, or a power greater than oneself

Defining characteristics:
Connections to self: desire to enhanced—hope, meaning and purpose in life, peace/serenity, acceptance, surrender, love, forgiveness of self, satisfying philosophy of life, joy, courage; heightened coping; meditation
Connections with others: provides service to others; requests interactions with spiritual leaders; requests forgiveness of others; requests interactions with friends, family
Connections with art, music, literature, nature: displays creative energy (e.g., writing, poetry); signs/listens to music; reads spiritual literature; spends time outdoors
Connections with power greater than self: prays; reports mystical experiences; participates in religious activities; expresses reverence, awe

Suffocation, risk for
Definition: accentuated risk of accidental suffocation (i.e., inadequate air available for inhalation)
Risk factors:
External: vehicle warming in closed garage; use of fuel-burning heaters not vented to outside; smoking in bed; children playing with plastic bags or inserting small objects into their mouths or noses; propped bottle placed in an infant's crib; pillow placed in an infant's crib; person who eats large mouthfuls of food; discarded or unused refrigerators or freezers without removed doors; children left unattended in bathtubs or pools; household gas leaks; low-strung clothesline; pacifier hung around infant's head
Internal: reduced olfactory sensation; reduced motor abilities; cognitive or emotional difficulties; disease or injury process; lack of safety education; lack of safety precautions

Suicide, risk for
Definition: at risk for self-inflicted, life-threatening injury
Risk factors:
Behavioral: history of prior suicide attempt; impulsiveness; buying a gun; stockpiling medicines; making or changing a will; giving away possessions; sudden euphoric recovery from major depression; marked change is in behavior, attitude, school performance
Verbal: threats of killing oneself; states desire to die/end it all
Situational: living alone; retired; relocation, institutionalization; economic instability; loss of autonomy/independence; presence of gun in home; adolescents living in nontraditional setting (e.g., juvenile detention center, prison, half-way house, group home)
Psychological: family history of suicide; alcohol and substance use/abuse; psychiatric illness/disorder (e.g., depression, schizophrenia, bipolar disorder); abuse in childhood; guilt; gay or lesbian youth
Demographic: age: elderly, young adult males, adolescents; race: Caucasian, Native American; gender: male; divorced, widowed
Physical: physical illness; terminal illness; chronic pain
Social: loss of important relationship; disrupted family life; grief, bereavement; poor support systems; loneliness; hopelessness; helplessness; social isolation; legal or disciplinary problem; cluster suicides

Surgical recovery, delayed
Definition: extension of the number of postoperative days required for individuals to initiate and perform on their own behalf activities that maintain life, health, and well-being

Related factors: to be developed
Defining characteristics: evidence of interrupted healing of surgical area (e.g., red, indurated, draining, immobile); loss of appetite with or without nausea; difficulty in moving about; requires help to complete self-care; fatigue; report of pain/discomfort; postpones resumption of work/employment activities; perception more time is needed to recover

Swallowing, impaired
Definition: abnormal functioning of the swallowing mechanism associated with deficits in oral, pharyngeal, or esophageal structure or function
Related factors:
Congenital deficits: upper airway anomalies; failure to thrive or protein energy malnutrition; conditions with significant hypotonia; respiratory disorders; history of tube feeding; behavioral feeding problems; self injurious behavior; neuromuscular impairment (e.g., decreased or absent gag reflex, decreased strength or excursion of muscles involved in mastication, perceptual impairment, facial paralysis); mechanical obstruction (e.g., edema, tracheostomy tube, tumor); congenital heart disease; cranial nerve involvement
Neurological problems: upper airway anomalies; laryngeal abnormalities; achalasia; gastroesophageal reflux disease; acquired anatomic defects; cerebral palsy; internal traumas; tracheal, laryngeal, esophageal defects; traumatic head injury; developmental delay; external traumas; nasal or nasopharyngeal cavity defects; oral cavity or oropharynx abnormalities; premature infants
Defining characteristics:
Pharyngeal phase impairment: altered head positions; inadequate laryngeal elevation; food refusal; unexplained fevers; delayed swallow; recurrent pulmonary infections; gurgly voice quality; nasal reflux; choking, coughing, or gagging; multiple swallows; abnormality in pharyngeal phase by swallow study
Esophageal phase impairment: heartburn or epigastric pain; acidic smelling breath; unexplained irritability surrounding mealtime; vomitus on pillow; repetitive swallowing or ruminating; regurgitation of gastric contents or wet burps; bruxism; nighttime coughing or awakening; observed evidence of difficulty in swallowing (e.g., stasis of food in oral cavity, coughing/choking); hyperextension of head, arching during or after meals; abnormality in esophageal phase by swallow study; odynophagia; food refusal or volume limiting; complaints of "something stuck"; hematemesis; vomiting
Oral phase impairment: lack of tongue action to form bolus; weak suck resulting in inefficient nippling; incomplete lip closure; food pushed out of mouth; slow bolus formation; food falls from mouth; premature entry of bolus; nasal reflux; inability to clear oral cavity; long meals with little consumption; coughing, choking, gagging before a swallow; abnormality in oral phase of swallow study; piecemeal deglutition; lack of chewing; pooling lateral sulci; sialorrhea or drooling

Therapeutic regime, effective management of
Definition: pattern of regulating and integrating into daily living a program for treatment of illness and its sequelae that is satisfactory for meeting specific health goals
Related factors: to be developed
Defining characteristics: appropriate choices of daily activities for meeting the goals of a treatment or prevention program; illness symptoms are within a normal range of expectation; verbalized desire to manage the treatment of illness and prevention of sequelae; verbalized intent to reduce risk factors for progression of illness and sequelae

Therapeutic regime, ineffective management of
Definition: pattern of regulating and integrating into daily living a program for treatment of illness and the sequelae of illness that is unsatisfactory for meeting specific health goals
Related factors: perceived barriers; social support deficits; powerlessness; perceived susceptibility; perceived benefits; mistrust of regime and/or health care personnel; knowledge deficits; family patterns of health care; family conflict; excessive demands made on individual or family; economic difficulties; decisional conflicts; complexity of therapeutic regime; complexity of health care system; perceived seriousness; inadequate number and types of cues to action
Defining characteristics: choices of daily living ineffective for meeting the goals of a treatment or prevention program; verbalized desire to manage the treatment of illness and prevention of sequelae; verbalized that did not take action to reduce risk factors for progression of illness and sequelae; verbalized difficulty with regulation/integration of one or more prescribed regimens for treatment of illness and its effects or prevention of complications; acceleration of illness symptoms; verbalized that did not take action to include treatment regimens in daily routines

Therapeutic regime, readiness for enhanced
Definition: a pattern of regulating and integrating into daily living a program(s) for treatment of illness and its sequelae that is sufficient for meeting health-related goals and can be strengthened
Defining characteristics: expresses desire to manage the treatment of illness and prevention of sequelae; choices of daily living are appropriate for meeting the goals of treatment or prevention; expresses little to no difficulty with regulation/integration of one or more prescribed regimes for treatment of illness or prevention of complications; describes reduction of risk factors for progression of illness and sequelae; no unexpected acceleration of illness symptoms

Therapeutic regime, ineffective community management of
Definition: pattern of regulating and integrating into community processes programs for treatment and integrating into community processes programs for treatment of illness and the sequelae of illness that are unsatisfactory for meeting health-related goals
Related factors: to be developed
Defining characteristics: illness symptoms above the norm expected for the number and type of population; unexpected acceleration of illness(es); number of health care resources are insufficient for the incidence or prevalence of illness(es); deficits in people and programs to be accountable for illness care of aggregates; deficits in community activities for secondary and tertiary prevention; deficits in advocates for aggregates; unavailable health care resources for illness care

Therapeutic regime, ineffective family management of
Definition: pattern of regulating and integrating into family processes a program for treatment of illness and the sequelae of illness that is unsatisfactory for meeting specific health goals
Related factors: complexity of health care system; complexity of therapeutic regime; decisional conflicts; economic difficulties; excessive demands made on individual or family; family conflict
Defining characteristics: inappropriate family activities for meeting the goals of a treatment or prevention program; acceleration of illness symptoms of a family member; lack of attention to illness and its sequelae; verbalize difficulty with regulation/integration of one or more effects or prevention of

complication; verbalized desire to manage the treatment of illness and prevention of the sequelae; verbalizes that family did not take action to reduce risk factors for progression of illness and sequelae

Thermoregulation, ineffective
Definition: temperature fluctuates between hypothermia and hyperthermia
Related factors: aging; fluctuating environmental temperature; immaturity; trauma or illness
Defining characteristics: fluctuations in body temperature above or below the normal range; cool skin; cyanotic nail beds; flushed skin; hypertension; increased respiratory rate; pallor (moderate); piloerection; reduction in body temperature below normal range; seizures/convulsions; shivering (mild); slow capillary refill; tachycardia; warm to touch

Thought processes, disturbed
Definition: disruption in cognitive operations and activities
Related factors: to be developed
Defining characteristics: cognitive dissonance; memory deficit/problems; inaccurate interpretation of environment; hypovigilance; hypervigilance; distractibility; egocentricity; inappropriate nonreality-based thinking

Tissue integrity, impaired
Definition: damage to mucous membrane, corneal, integumentary, or subcutaneous tissues
Related factors: mechanical (e.g., pressure, shear, friction); radiation (including therapeutic radiation); nutritional deficit or excess; thermal (temperature extremes); knowledge deficit; irritants, chemical (including body excretions, secretions, medications); impaired physical mobility; altered circulation; fluid deficit or excess.
Defining characteristics: damaged or destroyed tissue (e.g., cornea, mucous membrane, integumentary, or subcutaneous)

Tissue perfusion, ineffective (specify type: renal, cerebral, cardiopulmonary, gastrointestinal, peripheral)
Definition: decrease in oxygen resulting in the failure to nourish the tissues at the capillary level
Related factors: hypovolemia; interruption of flow, arterial; hypervolemia; exchange problems; interruption of flow, venous; mechanical reduction of venous and/or arterial blood flow; hypoventilation; impaired transport of the oxygen across alveolar and/or capillary membrane; mismatch of ventilation with blood flow; decreased hemoglobin concentration in blood; enzyme poisoning; altered affinity of hemoglobin for oxygen
Defining characteristics:
Renal: altered blood pressure outside of acceptable parameters; hematuria; oliguria or anuria; elevation in blood urea nitrogen (BUN)/creatinine ratio; skin color diminished arterial pulsations; skin color pale on elevation, color does not return on lowering of leg; slow healing of lesions; claudication; blood pressure changes in extremities; bruits
Gastrointestinal: hypoactive or absent bowel sounds; nausea; abdominal distention; abdominal pain or tenderness
Peripheral: edema; positive Homan's sign; altered skin characteristics (hair, nails, moisture); weak or absent pulses; skin discolorations; skin temperature changes; *altered sensations*

Cerebral: speech abnormalities; changes in pupillary reactions; extremity weakness or paralysis; altered mental status; difficulty in swallowing; changes in motor response; behavioral changes

Cardiopulmonary: altered respiratory rate outside of acceptable parameters; use of accessory muscles; capillary refill greater than three seconds; abnormal arterial blood gases; chest pain; sense of "impending doom"; bronchospasms; dyspnea; arrhythmias; nasal flaring; chest retraction

Transfer ability, impaired

Definition: limitation of independent movement between two nearby surfaces (specify level)

Suggested Functional Level Classification:

0 = is completely independent

1 = requires use of equipment or device

2 = requires help from another person for assistance, supervision, or teaching

3 = requires help from another person and equipment/device

4 = is dependent; does not participate in activity

Related factors: to be developed

Defining characteristics: impaired ability to transfer from bed to chair and chair to bed; impaired ability to transfer on or off a toilet or commode; impaired ability to transfer in and out of tub or shower; impaired ability to transfer from chair to car or car to chair; impaired ability to transfer from chair to floor or floor to chair; impaired ability to transfer from standing to floor or floor to standing

Trauma, risk for

Definition: accentuated risk of accidental tissue injury (e.g., wound, burn, fracture)

Risk factors:

External: high crime neighborhood and vulnerable clients; pot handles facing toward front of stove; knives stored uncovered; inappropriate call-for-aid mechanisms for bed-resting client; inadequately stored combustible or corrosives (e.g., matches, oily rags, lye); highly flammable children's toys or clothing; obstructed passageways; high beds; large icicles hanging from roof; nonuse or misuse of seat restraints; overexposure to sun, sun lamps, radiotherapy; overloaded electrical outlets; overloaded fuse boxes; play or work near vehicle pathways (e.g., driveways, laneways, railroad tracks); playing with fireworks or gunpowder; guns or ammunition stored unlocked; contact with rapidly moving machinery, industrial belts, or pulleys; litter or liquid spills on floors or stairways; defective appliances; bathing in very hot water (e.g., unsupervised bathing of young children); bathtub without hand grip or antislip equipment; children playing with matches, candles, cigarettes, sharp-edged toys; children riding in the front seat in car; delayed lighting of gas burner or oven; contact with intense cold; grease waste collected on stoves; driving a mechanically unsafe vehicle; driving after partaking of alcoholic beverages or drugs; driving at excessive speeds; entering unlighted rooms; experimenting with chemical or gasoline; exposure to dangerous machinery; faulty electrical plugs; frayed wires; contact with acids or alkalis; unsturdy or absent stair rails; use of unsteady ladders or chairs; use of cracked dishware or glasses; wearing plastic apron or flowing clothes around open flame; unscreened fires or heaters; unsafe window protection in homes with young children; sliding on coarse bed linen or struggling within bed restraints; use of thin or worn potholders; misuse of necessary headgear for motorized cyclists or young children carried on adult bicycles; potential igniting gas leaks; unsafe road or road-crossing conditions; slippery floors (e.g., wet or highly waxed); smoking in bed or near oxygen; snow or ice collected on stairs, walkways; unanchored electric wires; unanchored rugs, driving without necessary visual aids

Internal: lack of safety education; insufficient finances to purchase safety equipment or effect repairs; history of previous trauma; lack of safety precautions; poor vision; reduced temperature and/or tactile sensation; balancing difficulties; cognitive or emotional difficulties; reduced large or small muscle coordination; weakness; reduced hand-eye coordination

Urinary elimination, altered
Definition: disturbance in urine elimination
Related factors: urinary tract infection; anatomical obstruction; multiple causality; sensory motor impairment
Defining characteristics: incontinence; urgency; nocturia; hesitancy; frequency; dysuria; retention

Urinary elimination, readiness for enhanced
Definition: a pattern of urinary functions that is sufficient for meeting eliminatory needs and can be strengthened
Defining characteristics: expresses willingness to enhance urinary elimination; urine is straw colored with no odor; specific gravity is within normal limits; amount of output is within normal limits for age and other factors; positions self for emptying of bladder; fluid intake is adequate for daily needs

Urinary retention
Definition: incomplete emptying of bladder
Related factors: blockage; high urethral pressure caused by weak detrusor; inhibition of reflex arc; strong sphincter
Defining characteristics: bladder distention; small, frequent voiding or absence of urine output; dribbling; dysuria; overflow incontinence; residual urine; sensation of bladder fullness

Ventilation, impaired spontaneous
Definition: decreased energy reserves results in an individual's inability to maintain breathing adequate to support life
Related factors: respiratory muscle fatigue; metabolic factors
Defining characteristics: dyspnea; increased metabolic rate; increased pCO_2; increased restlessness; increased heart rate; decreased tidal volume; decreased pO_2; decreased cooperation; apprehension; decreased SaO_2; increased use of accessory muscles

Ventilatory weaning response, dysfunctional
Definition: inability to adjust to lowered levels of mechanical ventilator support that interrupts and prolongs the weaning process
Related factors:
Psychological: patient perceived inefficacy about the ability to wean; powerlessness; anxiety: moderate to severe; knowledge deficit of the weaning process; patient role; hopelessness; fear; decreased motivation; decreased self-esteem; insufficient trust in the nurse
Situational: uncontrolled episodic energy demands or problems; adverse environment (e.g., noisy, active environment, negative events in the room, low nurse-patient ratio, extended nurse absence from bedside, unfamiliar nursing staff); history of multiple unsuccessful weaning attempts; history of

ventilator dependence greater than 1 week; inappropriate pacing of diminished ventilator support; inadequate social support.

Defining characteristics:

Severe: deterioration in arterial blood gases from current baseline; respiratory rate increases significantly from baseline; increase from baseline blood pressure (>20 mm Hg); agitation; increase from baseline heart rate (>20 beats/min); paradoxical abdominal breathing; adventitious breath sounds, audible airway secretions; cyanosis; decreased level of consciousness; full respiratory accessory muscle use; shallow, gasping breaths; profuse diaphoresis; discoordinated breathing with the ventilator

Moderate: slight increase from baseline blood pressure (<20 mm Hg); baseline increase in respiratory rate (<5 breaths/min); slight increase from baseline heart rate (<20 beats/min); pale, slight cyanosis; slight respiratory accessory muscle use; inability to respond to coaching; inability to cooperate; apprehension; color changes; decreased air entry on auscultation; diaphoresis; eye widening (wide-eyed look); hypervigilance to activities

Mild: warmth; restlessness; slight increase of respiratory rate from baseline; queries about possible machine malfunction; expressed feelings of increased need for oxygen; fatigue; increased concentration on breathing; breathing discomfort

Violence, risk for other-directed

Definition: at risk for behaviors in which an individual demonstrates that he/she can be physically, emotionally, and/or sexually harmful to others

Risk factors: history of violence against others (e.g., hitting someone, kicking someone, spitting at someone, biting someone, attempted rape, rape, sexual molestation, urinating/defecating on a person); history of violence of threats (e.g., verbal threats against property, verbal threats against person, social threats, cursing, threatening notes/letters, threatening gestures, sexual threats); history of violent anti-social behavior (e.g., stealing, insistent borrowing, insistent demands for privileges, insistent interruption of meetings, refusal to eat, refusal to take medication, ignoring instructions); history of violence, indirect (e.g., tearing off clothes, ripping objects off walls, writing on walls, urinating on floor, defecating on floor, stamping feet, temper tantrum, running in corridors, yelling, throwing objects, breaking a window, slamming doors, sexual advances); other factors: neurological impairment (e.g., positive EEG, CAT, or MRI, head trauma, positive neurological findings, seizure disorders); cognitive impairment (e.g., learning disabilities, attention deficit disorder, decreased intellectual functioning); history of childhood abuse; history of witnessing family violence; cruelty to animals; firesetting; prenatal and perinatal complications/abnormalities; history of drug/alcohol abuse; pathological intoxication; psychotic symptomatology (e.g., auditory, visual, command hallucinations; paranoid delusions; loose, rambling of illogical thought processes); motor vehicle offenses (e.g., frequent traffic violations, use of a motor vehicle to release anger); suicidal behavior, impulsivity; availability and/or possession of weapon(s); body language; rigid posture, clenching of fists and jaw, hyperactivity, pacing, breathlessness, threatening stances.

Violence, risk for self-directed

Definition: at risk for behaviors in which an individual demonstrates that he/she can be physically, emotionally and/or sexually harmful to self

Risk factors: age 15–19; age over 45; marital status (single, widowed, divorced); employment (unemployed, recent job loss/failure); occupation (executive, administrator/owner of business, professional, semi-skilled worker); conflictual interpersonal relationships; family background (chaotic or conflictual, history of suicide); sexual orientation (bisexual [active], homosexual [inactive]); physical health (hypochondriac, chronic or terminal illness); mental health (severe depression, psychosis, severe personality disorder, alcoholism or drug abuse); emotional status (hopelessness, despair, increased anxiety, panic, anger, hostility); history of multiple suicide attempts; suicidal ideation (frequent, intense, prolonged); suicidal plan (clear and specific; lethality: method and availability of destructive means); personal resources (poor achievement, poor insight, affect unavailable and poorly controlled); social resources (poor rapport, socially isolated, unresponsive family); verbal clues (e.g., talking about death, "better off without me", asking questions about lethal dosages of drugs); behavioral clues (e.g., writing forlorn love notes, directing angry messages at a significant other who has rejected the person, giving away personal items, taking out a large life insurance policy); people who engage in autoerotic sexual acts

Walking, impaired
Definition: limitation of independent movement within the environment on foot (specify level)
Suggested Functional Level Classification:
0 = is completely independent
1 = requires use of equipment or device
2 = requires help from another person for assistance, supervision, or teaching
3 = requires help from another person and equipment/device
4 = is dependent; does not participate in activity
Related factors: to be developed
Defining characteristics: impaired ability to climb stairs; impaired ability to walk required distances; impaired ability to walk on an incline or decline; impaired ability to walk on uneven surfaces; impaired ability to navigate curbs

Wandering
Definition: meandering, aimless or repetitive locomotion that exposes the individual to harm; frequently incongruent with boundaries, limits, or obstacles
Related factors: cognitive impairment, specifically memory and recall deficits, disorientation, poor visuoconstructive (or visuospatial) ability, language (primarily expressive) deficits; cortical atrophy; premorbid behavior (e.g., outgoing, sociable personality, premorbid dementia); separation from familiar people and places; sedation; emotional state, especially frustration, anxiety, boredom, or depression (agitation); over/under-stimulating social or physical environment; physiological state of need (e.g., hunger, thirst, pain, urination, constipation); time of day
Defining characteristics: frequent or continuous movement from place to place, often revisiting the same destinations; persistent locomotion in search of "missing" or unattainable people or places; haphazard locomotion; locomotion into unauthorized or private places; locomotion resulting in unintended leaving of a premise; long periods of locomotion without an apparent destination; fretful locomotion or pacing; inability to locate significant landmarks in a familiar setting; locomotion that cannot be easily dissuaded or redirected; following behind or shadowing a caregiver's locomotion; trespassing; hyperactivity; scanning, seeking, or searching behaviors; periods of locomotion interspersed with periods of nonlocomotion (e.g., sitting, standing, sleeping); getting lost

Appendix B
SAMPLE DATA COLLECTION TOOLS AND DOCUMENTATION FORMS

INVASIVE PROCEDURES	DATE	SITE	DATE	RESPIRATORY THERAPY	MEDICATIONS	DOSAGE	METHOD	INTERVAL	HOURS
A LINE				TYPE					
SWAN-GANZ				O₂					
CVP LINE									
TRIPLE LUMEN									
®ATRIAL CATHETER									
PORTACATH									
NG TUBE									
SHUNT / ACCESS				DIAGNOSTICS					
WOUND DRAIN #1				I & Oq					
WOUND DRAIN #2				C & Aq					
URINARY CATHETER				FUNDAL /q					
CHEST TUBE #1				DTR'Sq					
CHEST TUBE #2				LOCHIA /q					
PACEMAKER P/T									
FIXED / DEMAND									
V / A-V SEQ.				ACTIVITIES					
OUTPUT				CBR					
PACING THRESHOLD				BRP					
SENS. RATE				AMB					
A / V INT.				W/C					
TRACHEOSTOMY / SIZE				TCDBq					
DIALYSIS H/P				POSITIONING					
COLOSTOMY				ROMq					

IV THERAPY

FLUID / TYPE	RATE / HR.	SITE	DATE INS.	DRESSING CHANGE	TUBING CHANGE	INSERTION SITE CHANGE

START DATE	PRN MEDICATION

DATE	NURSING TREATMENTS AND SPECIAL PROCEDURES

DATE	VITAL SIGNS
	TPRq
	BPq
	NEURO /q

DATE	TREATMENTS
	SITZ BATH
	TED HOSE

DATE	SPECIAL NEEDS
	ORIENTED
	DISORIENTED/HIGH RISK
	R/O PPD
	SUICIDE PRECAUTIONS
	SEIZURE PRECAUTIONS

KARDEX REVIEWED PRIOR TO TRANSFER

BY DR.	DATE
SIGNATURE	
BY DR.	DATE
SIGNATURE	
BY DR.	DATE
SIGNATURE	

APPENDIX B–1 The Kardex is a quick reference tool, sometimes used during report. Reprinted with permission from Conroe Regional Medical Center Hospital, Conroe, Texas.

(continues)

(continued)

SUNDAY	DATE	MONDAY	DATE	TUESDAY	DATE	WEDNESDAY	DATE

THURSDAY	DATE	FRIDAY	DATE	SATURDAY	DATE	DAILY & TIMED

COMMUNICATIONS

ISOLATION: TYPE _____

HIGH-RISK PATIENT YES ☐ NO ☐

NOTIFY IN EMERGENCY

NAME	RELATIONSHIP	ADDRESS	PHONE NO.

MONITOR	CODE BLUE	DATE	D.N.R.	DATE	PER:	PHYSICIAN

ALLERGIES

DIET	HEIGHT	WEIGHT
SURGERY		DATE

DATE OF ADMIT	DIAGNOSIS	SEX	AGE	PRIMARY PHYSICIAN

ROOM NO. | PATIENTS NAME

NS-34 (REV. 9/86) | CONSULTS

GEST_____ GR_____ PARA_____ AB_____ ANESTH_____

EPIS_____ LAC_____ RUBELLA IMMUNE/NON-IMMUNE_____

MOTHERS BLOOD TYPE_____ RH_____ BOTTLE/BREAST_____

BABYS BLOOD TYPE_____ WT_____ SEX_____ APGAR_____

DELIVERY DATE_____ TIME_____

Patient History and General Information ☐ ID bracelet placed

Nursing Unit: _____ Date: _____ Time: _____ Mode: ☐ Ambulatory ☐ Wheelchair ☐ Stretcher ☐ Ambulance
Origin: ☐ Home ☐ Dr's Office ☐ ER ☐ Nursing Home ☐ Other_____ Marital Status: ☐ Single ☐ Married ☐ Divorced ☐ Widowed
Information Provided by ☐ Patient ☐ Family/SO_____ ☐ No Available Informant at Time of Admission ☐ Transfer Form

GENERAL

Chief complaint / Reason for hospitalization: (State in patient's own words) _____
Summarize current illness episode _____

Initial vital signs   T_____ P_____ R_____   BP: RA _____ LA _____   Height: _____
☐ TYMPANIC ☐ ORAL ☐ RECTAL ☐ AXILLARY   ☐ LYING ☐ STANDING ☐ SITTING   Weight: stated_____ actual_____

MEDICAL HISTORY

Family History
☐ Diabetes ☐ Asthma ☐ COPD ☐ Heart Disease ☐ High BP ☐ Cancer ☐ Kidney Disease ☐ Seizures
Patient History
☐ Diabetes ☐ Asthma ☐ COPD ☐ Heart Disease ☐ High BP ☐ Cancer ☐ Kidney Disease ☐ Seizures ☐ Hepatitis ☐ Glaucoma
Other medical and surgical history _____

Patient Allergy History   ☐ No Known Allergies   ☐ If Allergy bracelet placed
☐ Food _____
☐ Medications _____
☐ Latex (Rubber) _____
☐ Dyes/Contrast Media _____
☐ Other _____
☐ Anesthesia Reaction _____   ☐ Transfusion Reaction _____

☐ Potential for Injury, Allergy
☐ Activate Latex Avoidance Practices

CURRENT MEDICATIONS

Name / Dose / Time *Include Herbs and Botanicals*	Last Dose	Code	Name / Dose / Time *Include Herbs and Botanicals*	Last Dose	Code	CODES
						A - Sent home with family
						B - At Bedside
						C - Not Brought with Patient
						D - In Pharmacy
						☐ Pt. instructed not to take own meds

Tobacco / Drug Usage   Alcohol Consumption

VALUABLES

	Home	Safe	Pt	N/A		Home	Safe	Pt	N/A
Wallet	☐	☐	☐	☐	Prosthesis	☐	☐	☐	☐
$	☐	☐	☐	☐	Jewelry	☐	☐	☐	☐
Artificial Eye	☐	☐	☐	☐	Clothing	☐	☐	☐	☐
Hearing Aid	☐	☐	☐	☐	Wheelchair	☐	☐	☐	☐
Glasses	☐	☐	☐	☐	Cane/Walker	☐	☐	☐	☐
Contacts	☐	☐	☐	☐	Brace	☐	☐	☐	☐
Upper Dent.	☐	☐	☐	☐	Crutches	☐	☐	☐	☐
Lower Dent.	☐	☐	☐	☐	Other	☐	☐	☐	☐

Patient / SO acknowledges that Conroe Regional Medical Center shall not be liable for loss or damage of any money, jewelry, documents, clothing or other personal property of patients or visitors unless deposited for safekeeping in the hospital safe.

Patient Signature _____
Staff Signature _____

Date _____ Time _____
Data Collector's Signature _____ RN/LVN

PATIENT ORIENTATION TO ENVIRONMENT

Equipment Instructions:
☐ Bed ☐ Call Light ☐ Phone ☐ Temp Control ☐ Siderails
☐ TV ☐ Monitors ☐ IV Pump ☐ O2 Safety ☐ Admit Kit
☐ Bathroom Call Light ☐ Mealtimes ☐ Isolation Procedures (if applicable)
Rights and Responsibilities Instructions:
☐ Smoking Policy & Areas ☐ Visiting Hours ☐ Patient Handbook

RIGHTS AND RESPONSIBILITIES

☐ Patient has a Directive to Physician / Medical Power of Attorney
___ Copy is on front of chart
___ Requested to provide the hospital with a copy
☐ Advance Directive Follow up Copy

Medical Power of Attorney Name   Tele #

☐ Patient has not executed an Advance Directive
___ Patient handbook info provided / discussed in registration
___ Patient handbook info provided / discussed on the unit
___ Patient wants assistance to execute one
☐ Advance Directive Follow up Execute

☐ Patient unable / unwilling to discuss at time of admission to the unit
☐ Family unavailable at time of admission to the unit
☐ Advance Directive Follow up Info

PATIENT IDENTIFICATION

Conroe Regional Medical Center

ADMISSION ASSESSMENT

NS-102 (REV. 02/00)

(continues)

APPENDIX B-2 Admission Assessment Form.
Reprinted with permission from Conroe Regional Medical Center Hospital, Conroe, Texas.

(continued)

Biophysical Psychosocial Assessment (completed by RN)

NORM	VARIANCE	PATIENT PROBLEM / NSG DIAGNOSIS
Neurological Assessment Alert and oriented to person, place and time. Behavior appropriate to situation. Pupils equal and reactive to light. Active ROM of all extremities and symmetry of strength. No Parasthesia. ☐ ALL PARAMETERS WNL	DISORIENTED ☐ Time ☐ Person ☐ Place PUPILS ☐ Non Reactive R__ L __ ☐ Sluggish R__ L __ ☐ Unequal ☐ Pinpoint R__ L __ ☐ Dilated R__ L __ SENSORY MOTOR IMPAIRMENT ☐ Speech ☐ Swallowing ☐ Visual ☐ Headaches ☐ Seizures ☐ Gait disturbance ☐ Unequal hand grasp ☐ Numbness ☐ Tingling	☐ Confusion ☐ Acute ☐ Chronic ☐ Thought Processes, alteration ☐ Communication, impaired, verbal ☐ Swallowing, impaired ☐ Peripheral Neurovascular, alteration ☐ Tissue Perfusion, alteration ☐ Sensory Perception, alteration
Cardiovascular Assessment Regular Radial pulse. Capillary Refill Time < 3 sec. Peripheral pulses palpable. No edema. No calf tenderness. ☐ ALL PARAMETERS WNL	☐ Rhythm irregular ☐ Tachycardia > 100 ☐ Bradycardia < 60 ☐Telemetry Number _____Rhythm BP_____ ☐ Hypertension ☐ Hypotension ☐ Chest Pain EDEMA ☐ Feet/Ankles R__ L __ ☐ Pitting + _____ PULSES ☐ Abnormal Location _____	☐ Activity, intolerance ☐ Fluid Volume, deficit ☐ Fluid Volume, excess ☐ Tissue Perfusion, alteration ☐
Respiratory Assessment Regular, non labored. Breath sounds clear and equal all lobes. Respirations 12 - 20 per minute. Sputum clear, nailbeds and mucus membranes pink. ☐ ALL PARAMETERS WNL	COUGH ☐ Non Productive ☐ Sputum _____ BREATH SOUNDS ☐ Diminished R__ L __ ☐ Rhonchi R__L __ ☐ Wheezes R__ L__ ☐ Crackles R__ L __ ☐ Dyspnea ☐ Apnea ☐ Tachypnea ___ ☐ Uneven Chest Movement ☐ ET Tube ☐ Trach ☐ Vent ☐ O2 Mask ☐ O2L ___ O2 Sat ___	☐ Airway Clearance, ineffective ☐ Breathing Pattern, ineffective ☐ Tissue Perfusion, alteration ☐
Gastrointestinal Assessment Abdomen soft, non distended, non tender. Bowel sounds present in 4 quadrants. Bowel movements within own normal patterns and consistency. ☐ ALL PARAMETERS WNL	BOWEL SOUNDS ☐ Absent ☐ Hypoactive ☐ Hyperactive COMPLAINTS ☐ Constipation ☐ Flatus ☐ Nausea ☐ Vomiting ☐ Increased Thirst ☐ Laxative Dependence ABDOMEN ☐ Distended ☐ Tender ☐ Rebound ☐ Hard TUBES ☐ NGT ☐ Feeding Tube ☐JP Drain ☐ Hernovac ☐ Tube ☐ Gastrojejunostomy ☐ Colostomy ☐ Ileostomy ☐ Other_____	☐ Bowel Elimination, alteration ☐ Diarrhea ☐ Constipation ☐ Incontinence ☐ Nutrition, alteration ☐ Tissue Perfusion, alteration ☐
Integumentary Assessment Skin color uniform within patient's norm. Smooth, soft, warm, dry, intact. Turgor skin lifts easily and snaps back immediately on release. Mucus membranes moist, intact, pink. Hygiene good. ☐ ALL PARAMETERS WNL	SKIN APPEARANCE ☐ Pale ☐ Cyanotic ☐ Dusky ☐ Mottled ☐ Flushed ☐ Jaundiced ☐ Other ☐ Hygiene Inadequate SKIN TEMP / CHARACTER ☐ Hot ☐ Cold ☐ Clammy ☐ Moist ☐ Turgor Sluggish / Poor ☐ Very Dry MUCUS MEMBRANES ☐ Dry ☐ Blistered ☐ Cracking CONDITION ☐ Impairment (see Dermal Injury Section)	☐ Skin Integrity, Impaired ☐ Tissue Integrity, impaired ☐ Oral Mucus Membrane, alteration ☐ Body Temperature, alteration ☐ Tissue Perfusion, alteration ☐
Musculoskeletal Assessment Absence of joint swelling and tenderness. Normal ROM of all joints. No muscle weakness. Surrounding tissues show no evidence of inflammation, nodules, nail changes, ulcerations or rashes. No deformity. ☐ ALL PARAMETERS WNL	☐ Joint Swelling / Tenderness ☐ Immobile ☐Paralysis ☐ Deformity ☐ Atrophy ☐ Contracture HOMANS POSITIVE Right ☐ Absent Left ☐ Absent ☐ Present ☐ Present	☐ Physical Mobility, impaired ☐ Peripheral Neurovascular, alteration ☐ Tissue Perfusion, alteration ☐
Genitourinary Assessment Able to empty bladder without dysuria. Bladder not distended after voiding. Urine clear and yellow to amber. Continent of Urine. No appliances used. ☐ ALL PARAMETERS WNL	☐ Hemodialysis ☐ Peritoneal Dialysis ☐ Urostomy ☐ Foley # URINE Color____ ☐ Cloudy ☐ Sediment ☐ Frequency ☐ Burning ☐ Incontinent ☐ Bladder Distention / Retention ☐ Hematuria ☐ Nocturia ☐ Anuria ☐ In and Out Cath Pt ___ Family ___ _____	☐ Urinary Elimination, alteration ☐ Retention ☐ Incontinence ☐ Tissue Perfusion, alteration ☐
Reproductive / Sexuality If female, no vaginal bleeding, discharge or lesions. Normal menstrual periods. If male, no prostrate problems, penile bleeding, lesions or discharge. No complaints of sexual dysfunction. ☐ ALL PARAMETERS WNL	☐ Discharge color _____ amount _____ ☐ Unusual Bleeding ☐ Pain ☐ Diagnosis may affect sexuality ☐ Pregnant ☐ Post partum ☐ Breastfeeding _____	☐ Sexual dysfunction ☐ Sexual Pattern, impaired ☐ Body Image, disturbance ☐
Psycho / Social Assessment Behavior apropriate to situation. Cooperative congruent affect. Responds appropriately to all questions. ☐ ALL PARAMETERS WNL	☐ Flat Affect ☐ Lack of eye contact ☐ Withdrawn ☐Agitated ☐ Crying ☐ Uncooperative ☐ Anxious ☐ Irritable ☐ Nervous ☐ Combative ☐ Threatening ☐ Ineffective Grieving o Unable to Cope ☐ Family Issues / Dysfunction	☐ Anxiety, fear ☐ Coping, ineffective ☐ Grieving, anticipatory ☐ Powerlessness ☐

RN INITIALS

PATIENT IDENTIFICATION

Conroe
Regional Medical Center

ADMISSION ASSESSMENT

NS-102 p.2 (REV. 02/00)

(continues)

(continued)

Biophysical Psychosocial Assessment

	PATIENT PROBLEM/NSG DIAGNOSIS

Pain Assessment
Do you have pain now? ☐ Yes ☐ No
Have you had pain in the last several weeks or months? ☐ Yes ☐ No
If Yes, to any of the above questions fill in information below.
  1. Pain Location _____
  _____
  2. Pain Description ☐ Dull ☐ Sharp ☐ Cramping ☐ Other _____
  3. Pain Intensity Adult Pain Scale   <u>No Pain</u> 0 1 2 3 4 5 6 7 8 9 10 <u>Worst Pain</u>
  4. Duration ☐ Constant ☐ Intermittent ☐ Other _____
  5. What helps the pain _____
  _____
  6. What aggravates the pain _____
  _____
	☐ Pain
	☐ Pain, chronic
	☐

Activities of Daily Living Assessment **ADL Needs** Hygiene ☐ self ☐ assist ☐ dependent **Sensory Deficits** Activity ☐ self ☐ assist ☐ dependent ☐ Vision _____ Nutrition ☐ self ☐ assist ☐ dependent ☐ Hearing_____ Toileting ☐ self ☐ assist ☐ dependent ☐ Speech_____ Sleep ☐ sleeps well at night ☐ Other_____ ☐ does not sleep well What helps sleep?_____ **Assistive Device Use** ☐ Cane ☐ Walker ☐ Wheelchair ☐ Bedside Commode ☐ Prosthesis ☐ Other_____	☐ Self Care, deficit ☐ Physical Mobility, impaired ☐ Activity, intolerance ☐ Sleep Pattern, disturbance ☐ Sensory Perception, alteration ☐ Communication, impaired verbal ☐

Cultural Spiritual Assessment
1. Are there any spiritual, traditional, ethnic, or cultural practice that you need to be part of your care
  ☐ Yes ☐ No
2. Is there any way the hospital can assist you with your religious / spiritual practices
  ☐ Yes ☐ No
3. Would you like to be visited by the hospital chaplain ☐ Yes ☐ No
	☐ Spiritual, distress
	☐ Cultural, distress
	☐ Grieving, anticipatory
	☐
	
	Notify Chaplain
	Notification Initials _____

PATIENT AND FAMILY EDUCATION NEEDS / READINESS ASSESSMENT	

Information Provided by ☐ Patient ☐ Family / SO ☐ No Available Informant at Time of Admission
1. **Literacy / Level of Education** Can Read ☐ Yes ☐ No Can Write ☐ Yes ☐ No
  Highest Level of Education _____
2. **Language** ☐ English ☐ Spanish ☐Other_____ Proficient in English ☐ Yes ☐ No
  Translator needed ☐Yes ☐ No
3. **Learning Barriers** ☐ None Identified ☐ Language ☐ Memory ☐ Vision ☐ Hearing ☐ Emotional
  ☐ Ability to grasp concepts and respond ☐ Motor Skills Impairment ☐ Other _____
4. **Concerns / Needs** ☐ None Identified ☐ First hospital visit ☐ Access to community resources
  ☐ Financial concerns ☐ Religious considerations ☐ School age children education needs
  ☐ Other _____
5. **Motivation** ☐ Wants to learn ☐ Uninterested, distracted or uncooperative ☐ Denies need
  ☐ Other_____
6. **Methods** Patient/Family says they learn best by ☐ Reading booklets, information sheets
  ☐ One to one discussions ☐ Hands on practice
  ☐ Other/Explain _____
7. **Type of Education** Do you or your family need information about
  ☐ No information specified ☐ Disease process ☐ Activity ☐ Medical Devices / Equipment ☐ Diet
  ☐ Current Medications / Drug Food Interactions ☐ Other _____
	☐ Knowledge Deficit
	R/T _____
	
	☐ Noncompliance
	
	☐ Communication, impaired
	Language _____

RN INITIALS _____

Conroe _____
Regional Medical Center

PATIENT IDENTIFICATION

| ADMISSION ASSESSMENT |

(continues)

(continued)

Safety Risk Assessment

B = burn
C = contusion
D = decubitus
E = erytthema
I = incision
L = laceration
P = petechiae
R = rash
S = scar

Left Foot   **Right Foot**

	0	1	2	Score
Mobility	Independent	Required Assistance	Total Assistance	
Continence	Continent	Occasional Incontinence	Incontinent	
Nutrition	> 90% diet	50-90% diet	< 50% diet	
Skin Integrity	Intact	Stage I or II Pressure Sore	Stage III, IV or Multi-pressure Sore	
Old Pressure Sores/Scars	No old scars	Scars over 1 Bony Prominence	Scar over 2 Bony Prominence	
Contractures/ Fractures	No contractures or fractures	Contracture 1 Extremity or Fracture	Contracture >2 Extremities; Fracture Pelvis, Non-Healed Amputation	

Total _____

Risk for Dermal Injury

☐ Skin Integrity, impairment risk for score 2 or >

☐ Skin Integrity Impaired

Location _____
Description _____
_____
_____

Location _____
Description _____
_____

Location _____
Description _____
_____

Age
☐ Sixty Years of Age or Older — 2
Medications
<u>Anesthesia</u>, <u>Diuretics</u>, <u>Laxatives</u>, <u>Narcotics</u>, <u>CNS Depressants</u>, <u>Hypertensives</u>, <u>Insulin</u>
☐ Uses one or more no adverse effects — 1
☐ Uses one or more with adverse effects — 2
Mobility
☐ Exhibits pattern of gait disturbance — 5
☐ Needs assist to toilet or transfer to chair — 5
Mentation
☐ Unable to comprehend instruction, use the call button or ask for assistance — 10
☐ Unable to make purposeful decisions — 10
Sensory Deficits
☐ Has impaired hearing, sight or speech — 3
History of falling
☐ Hx of orthostatic hypotension or seizures — 5
☐ Other reason _____ — 5

Total _____

Risk for Fall

☐ Injury, potential for fall for score 4 or >

TB RISK

☐ Hemoptysis   ☐ Productive Cough > 3 wks   ☐ Night Sweats   ☐ Weight Loss / Fever   ☐ None
*If any of these symptoms Initiate Airborne Precautions and Alert MD for Follow up

Risk for TB

☐ Infection, potential TB

DOMESTIC VIOLENCE

1. Do you currently feel unsafe at home? ☐ Yes ☐ No Why?_____
2. Have you been afraid, threatened or injured by anyone within the last year? o Yes o No
3. Have you been hit, slapped, kicked, forced to engage in unwanted sexual acts, or otherwise hurt by someone in the last year? ☐ Yes ☐ No_____

Risk for Domestic Violence
☐ Activate Hospital Protocol
☐ Injury, potential for abuse

RN INITIALS

Conroe
Regional Medical Center

PATIENT IDENTIFICATION

ADMISSION ASSESSMENT

NS- 102 p.4 (REV.02/00)

(continues)

(continued)

Multidisciplinary Screens

		SCORE	
NUTRITION	Usual Diet _____		If score = or > 2
	☐ Difficulty with any of the following > 1 week		Notify Dietitian
	☐ Vomiting ☐ Diarrhea ☐ Swallowing ☐ Chewing / Unable to eat	2	
	☐ Unplanned weight loss > 10 lb. in past 4 months	8	
	☐ Diagnosis of malnutrition / malabsorption	8	Notification initials: ____
	☐ Surgery this admission or within the past 30 days if 65 years or older	2	
	☐ Patient / family request diet education related to patient's modified diet of:_____	1	
	TOTAL: _____		

		SCORE	
DIABETES	☐ New diagnosis IDDM	2	If score = or > 1
	☐ New diagnosis NIDDM	1	Notify Diabetes Educator
	☐ New insulin start	2	
	☐ Gestational	2	If score = or > than 2
	☐ Recurrent hypoglycemia	1	Request MD Order
	☐ DKA or HHNK	2	
	☐ Recurrent ER visits for DM	1	Notification initials: ____
	TOTAL: _____		

		SCORE	
SPEECH PATHOLOGY	If ☐ Onset of the below criteria is a result of this illness or within 30 days of admission	1	If score = or > than 2
	And any one or more of the following		Notify Speech Pathology
	☐ Difficulty in making self understood or difficulty in understanding others	1	
	☐ Patient/family reported or clinically observed choking or coughing while eating or drinking	1	
	☐ Patient/family reported or clinically observed change in voice quality/teary eyes/nasal drainage after eating	1	Notification initials: ____
	☐ Recent significant weight loss, dehydration or pneumonia	1	
	☐ New laryngectomy or tracheostomy	1	
	☐ Patient admitted with order for thickened liquids	1	
	TOTAL: _____		

		SCORE	
PT/OT	If ☐ The onset of the below criteria is a result of this illness or within 30 days of admission	1	If score = or > than 3
	☐ Patient / Family demonstrates potential ability to participate in rehab	1	Notify PT / OT
	And any one or more of the following		
	☐ Impaired functional mobility (gait transfer or bed mobility) and/or a potential for injury	1	
	☐ Difficulty in performing ADLs (feeding, dressing, grooming)	1	
	☐ Difficulty in management of pain / stress	1	Notification initials: ____
	☐ Patient/family could benefit from splinting, positional or equipment management	1	
	☐ Potential physical / occupational therapy related discharge needs	1	
	TOTAL: _____		

		SCORE	
DISCHARGE PLANNING	**Patient lives:** ☐ alone ☐ with spouse ☐ with other family		If score is < than 5
	☐ assisted / extended care facility_____		Notify Case Management in Meditech
	Who can help after discharge: Name: _____ Relationship: _____		
	Telephone #: _____		If score = or > than 5
			Notify Case Management in Meditech and
	Receiving these services ☐ Home Health - Agency:_____		voicemail Hotline (# on
	prior to admission: ☐ Durable Medical Equipment - Provider:_____		call schedule)
	☐ Hospice - Provider:_____		
	☐ Return to prior living situation unlikely	2	
	☐ Unable to identify any assistance for after discharge at this time	2	
	☐ Home Health Services and / or Durable Medical Equipment need anticipated at discharge	2	Notification initials:
	☐ Skilled Nursing Facility or Inpatient Rehabilitation anticipated at discharge	2	
	☐ Nursing Home Placement anticipated at discharge	2	☐ Complex Discharge
	☐ Food, Clothing or Shelter needs identified	2	Needs
	☐ Suspected Abuse or Neglect (follow hospital policy for reporting)	5	
	☐ Positive Drug Screen with delivery	5	
	☐ Desires an adoption plan	5	
	☐ Discharge anticipated in less than 72 yours with any of the above items checked	3	
	TOTAL: _____		

_____ DATE   _____ TIME   _____ ADMISSION   _____ RN SIGNATURE

PATIENT IDENTIFICATION

Conroe
Regional Medical Center

ADMISSION ASSESSMENT

Date of Discharge	Time of Discharge	Mode of Discharge		Accom. by:
		☐ Ambulatory ☐ Wheelchair ☐ Stretcher ☐ Ambulance		_____

Belongings sent with patient or family ☐ Yes ☐ No	Personal medications sent with patient or family ☐ Yes ☐ No	Prescription sent with patient ☐ Yes ☐ No	Temp	P	R	BP

Discharge Destination
☐ Home ☐ AMA ☐ Facility_____ ☐ Other_____

Transfer Information Sent
☐ Yes   ☐ No

Special Instructions

Patient Assessment and Health Status

	Yes	No			Yes	No			Yes	No
Afebrile_____	☐	☐	Hygiene:				Skin Intact_____		☐	☐
Able to Live Independently_____	☐	☐	Self Care_____	☐	☐	Eating Well_____		☐	☐
Pain Controlled_____	☐	☐	Assist_____	☐	☐	Adequate Hydration_____		☐	☐
Oriented_____	☐	☐	Total Care_____	☐	☐				
Appropriate Behavior_____	☐	☐	Adequate Elimination_____	☐	☐				
Functions Independently_____	☐	☐							

Additional Comments

	Nurse Signature	Date

Instructions

Diet
☐ No Restrictions

Activity
☐ No Restrictions

Special Equipment/Treatment
☐ No Restrictions

Discharge Medications (Name, Amount, Special Instructions)
  ☐ No Meds   ☐ Rx Given

Special Instructions/Discharge Summary

☐ Pt. or Caregiver given instructions about and counseled on potential for drug-food interactions.

Physician Follow-Up Appointment	Outpatient Visit

Referral
☐ None Required

I have received all personal belongings.
I have received a copy and understand the above instructions.

PATIENT IDENTIFICATION

_____
Signature/Responsible Party

_____
Physician/Nurse Signature   Date

Discharge Assessment/Instructions

N5411 07/98 (RC# 4602080)

APPENDIX B–3 Discharge Assessment Forms.
Reprinted with permission from Conroe Regional Medical Center Hospital, Conroe, Texas.

CONROE REGIONAL MEDICAL CENTER

PATIENT CARE RECORD - OBSERVATIONS

DATE: _____

PATIENT I.D. PLATE

VITAL SIGNS

HOURS	NEURO VITAL SIGNS					PULSES		OBSTETRICAL					IV	BP :00	HR :00	RESP :00	TEMP :00	BP :15	HR :15	RESP :15	TEMP :15	BP :30	HR :30	RESP :30	TEMP :30	BP :45	HR :45	RESP :45	TEMP :45
	GCS MOTOR	PUPILS ® Ⓛ	EXTREM. R.A. / R.L.	L.A. / L.L.		R.A. / R.L.	L.A. / L.L.	BREASTS	FUNDUS/PLACEMENT	LOCHIA	PERINEUM	SITE CHECK																		
7A																														
8A																														
9A																														
10A																														
11A																														
12N																														
1P																														
2P																														
3P																														
4P																														
5P																														
6P																														
7P																														
8P																														
9P																														
10P																														
11P																														
12M																														
1A																														
2A																														
3A																														
4A																														
5A																														
6A																														

GLASGOW COMA SCALE

Eyes	Open	Spontaneously	4	Best	Oriented and converses	5
		To verbal command	3	verbal	Disoriented and converses	4
		To pain	2	response	Inappropriate words	3
		No response	1		Incomprehensible sounds	2
					No response	1
Best motor response	To verbal command	Obeys	6			
	To painful stimulus	Localizes Pain	5			
		Flexion-Withdrawal	4			
		Flexion-abnormal (decorticate rigidity)	3			
		Extension (decerebrate rigidity)	2			
		No response	1			

PUPILS + Reactive − Nonreactive ± Sluggish

PUPIL GAUGE (MM) 2 3 4 5 6 7 8 9

EXTREMITIES

MOVEMENT	ABBREV.	STRENGTH	MOVEMENT	ABBREV.
VOLUNTARY	V	+STRONG	NONE	∅
COMMAND	C	−WEAK	DECORTICATE	Decor.
STIM/PURPOSEFUL	S	∅ABSENT	DECEREBRATE	Decer.
WITHDRAWS	W			

PULSES

A-ABSENT   W-WEAK   S-STRONG   D-DOPPLER

OBSTETRICAL LEGEND

BREAST:	S-SOFT	F-FIRM	E-ENGORGED
FUNDUS/PLACEMENT		S-SOFT	F-FIRM
LOCHIA:	S-SCANT	M-MODERATE	H-HEAVY
PERINEUM	C-CLEAN /		E-EDEMA

NS-49 (Rev. 5/95)

PAGE-1

(continues)

APPENDIX B–4 24-hour Progress Notes.
Reprinted with permission from Conroe Regional Medical Center Hospital, Conroe, Texas.

(continued)

PATIENT CARE RECORD

PATIENT-FAMILY TEACHING

TIME	PROBLEM #	PATIENT - FAMILY TEACHING	INITIAL

TIME	PROBLEM #	PSYCHOSOCIAL INTERVENTIONS / DC PLANNING	INITIAL

POST PARTUM ASSESSMENT (To be used on obstetrical patients only.)

DAY SHIFT	EVENING SHIFT	NIGHT SHIFT
R L	**R L**	**R L**
REFLEXES 1+ 2+ 3+ 4+ 1+ 2+ 3+ 4+	REFLEXES 1+ 2+ 3+ 4+ 1+ 2+ 3+ 4+	REFLEXES 1+ 2+ 3+ 4+ 1+ 2+ 3+ 4+
CLONUS ABSENT ☐ ABSENT ☐	CLONUS ABSENT ☐ ABSENT ☐	CLONUS ABSENT ☐ ABSENT ☐
PRESENT ____ BEATS PRESENT ____ BEATS	PRESENT ____ BEATS PRESENT ____ BEATS	PRESENT ____ BEATS PRESENT ____ BEATS
HOMANS ABSENT ☐ ABSENT ☐	HOMANS ABSENT ☐ ABSENT ☐	HOMANS ABSENT ☐ ABSENT ☐
PRESENT ☐ PRESENT ☐	PRESENT ☐ PRESENT ☐	PRESENT ☐ PRESENT ☐
BREASTS SEE ☐ **NOTES** SOFT, TENDER, ENGORGED, FISSURES	**BREASTS** SEE ☐ **NOTES** SOFT, TENDER, ENGORGED, FISSURES	**BREASTS** SEE ☐ **NOTES** SOFT, TENDER, ENGORGED, FISSURES
FUNDUS FIRM, BOGGY LEVEL _____ BLADDER _____	**FUNDUS** FIRM, BOGGY LEVEL _____ BLADDER _____	**FUNDUS** FIRM, BOGGY LEVEL _____ BLADDER _____
PERINEUM - HEMORRHOIDS EPISIOTOMY - CLEAN, INTACT SWELLING, INFLAMMATION, DRAINAGE, HEMATOMA ☐ SEE NOTES	**PERINEUM - HEMORRHOIDS** EPISIOTOMY - CLEAN, INTACT SWELLING, INFLAMMATION, DRAINAGE, HEMATOMA ☐ SEE NOTES	**PERINEUM - HEMORRHOIDS** EPISIOTOMY - CLEAN, INTACT SWELLING, INFLAMMATION, DRAINAGE, HEMATOMA ☐ SEE NOTES
LOCHIA - VAG. DRAINAGE SM. - MED. - LARGE SEROSA - RUBRA - ALBA ☐ SEE NOTES	**LOCHIA - VAG. DRAINAGE** SM. - MED. - LARGE SEROSA - RUBRA - ALBA ☐ SEE NOTES	**LOCHIA - VAG. DRAINAGE** SM. - MED. - LARGE SEROSA - RUBRA - ALBA ☐ SEE NOTES
FEEDING SEE BREAST - BOTTLE - FOD ☐ NOTES	FEEDING SEE BREAST - BOTTLE - FOD ☐ NOTES	FEEDING SEE BREAST - BOTTLE - FOD ☐ NOTES
ROOMING IN YES - NO	**ROOMING IN** YES - NO	**ROOMING IN** YES - NO
BONDING POSITIVE - NEGATIVE	**BONDING** POSITIVE - NEGATIVE	**BONDING** POSITIVE - NEGATIVE
SIGNATURE TIME	SIGNATURE TIME	SIGNATURE TIME

(continues)

(continued)

**SEE CARE PLAN
NURSING DIAGNOSIS:**

#		#		#	
	Airway Clearance, Ineffective		Grieving		Pain
	Anxiety		Home Maintenance Management, Impaired		Sensory/Perceptual Alt.
	Breathing Patterns, Ineffective		Hyperthermia		Skin Integrity, Impaired
	Cardiac Output, Decreased		Incontinence		Sleep Pattern Disturbance
	Communication, Impaired Verbal		Injury, High Risk for		Social Isolation
	Coping, Ineffective Individual		Knowledge Deficit		Thought Process, Altered
	Fatigue		Mobility, Impaired Physical		Tissue Perfusion, Alt.
	Fluid Vol., Alt. in		Nutrition, Alt. in		
	Gas Exchange, Impaired		Noncompliance		
					See Critical Pathway

TIME	PROB #	PT. OUTCOME / EVALUATION

INITIALS	SIGNATURES	INITIALS	SIGNATURES	INITIALS	SIGNATURES

(continues)

(continued)

NURSING INTERVENTION

		DAY / INITIAL	EVENING / INITIAL	NIGHT / INITIAL
D I E T		DIET: NPO REG. SOFT CLEAR LIQUID FULL LIQUIDS SPECIAL TYPE: _____ FEED SELF, ASST. TOTAL ____ % DIET TAKEN SNACKS:	DIET: NPO REG. SOFT CLEAR LIQUID FULL LIQUIDS SPECIAL TYPE: _____ FEED SELF, ASST. TOTAL ____ % DIET TAKEN SNACKS:	DIET: NPO REG. SOFT CLEAR LIQUID FULL LIQUIDS SPECIAL TYPE: _____ FEED SELF, ASST. TOTAL ____ % DIET TAKEN SNACKS:
H Y G I E N E	☐ BED BATH ☐ TUB ☐ SHOWER ☐ SITZ	☐ NA ☐ SELF ☐ ASSIST ☐ COMPLETE	☐ NA ☐ SELF ☐ ASSIST ☐ COMPLETE	☐ NA ☐ SELF ☐ ASSIST ☐ COMPLETE
	HAIR/SHAVE	☐ YES ☐ NO	☐ YES ☐ NO	☐ YES ☐ NO
	ORAL CARE	☐ SELF ☐ COMPLETE ☐ ASSIST	☐ SELF ☐ COMPLETE ☐ ASSIST	☐ SELF ☐ COMPLETE ☐ ASSIST
	SKIN CARE	☐ NA ☐ SELF ☐ EGG CRATE ☐ ASSIST ☐ COMPLETE	☐ NA ☐ SELF ☐ EGG CRATE ☐ ASSIST ☐ COMPLETE	☐ NA ☐ SELF ☐ EGG CRATE ☐ ASSIST ☐ COMPLETE
	FOLEY CATH. CARE	☐ YES ☐ N/A	☐ YES ☐ N/A	☐ YES ☐ N/A
	DECUBITUS CARE	☐ YES ☐ N/A	☐ YES ☐ N/A	☐ YES ☐ N/A
	LINEN CHANGE	☐ YES ☐ NO	☐ YES ☐ NO	☐ YES ☐ NO
A C T I V I T Y	TYPE OF ACTIVITY	☐ BED ☐ CHAIR ☐ W/C ☐ AMB. ☐ DANGLE ☐ BRP ☐ ROM	☐ BED ☐ CHAIR ☐ W/C ☐ AMB. ☐ DANGLE ☐ BRP ☐ ROM	☐ BED ☐ CHAIR ☐ W/C ☐ AMB. ☐ DANGLE ☐ BRP ☐ ROM
	HOW ACCOMPLISHED	☐ SELF ☐ ASSIST ☐ PT ☐ WALKER ☐ CANE ☐ CRUTCH	☐ SELF ☐ ASSIST ☐ PT ☐ WALKER ☐ CANE ☐ CRUTCH	☐ SELF ☐ ASSIST ☐ PT ☐ WALKER ☐ CANE ☐ CRUTCH
	DEEP BREATHE AND COUGH	☐ Q2H ASSIST ☐ Q2H SELF @ ☐ IS@ ☐ N/A	☐ Q2H ASSIST ☐ Q2H SELF @ ☐ IS@ ☐ N/A	☐ Q2H ASSIST ☐ Q2H SELF @ ☐ IS@ ☐ N/A
	REST PERIOD POSITION/	☐ YES ☐ N/A ☐ Q2H ASSIST ☐ Q2H SELF @	☐ YES ☐ N/A ☐ Q2H ASSIST ☐ Q2H SELF @	
	REPOSITION	@ ☐ N/A	@ ☐ N/A	@ ☐ N/A
T R E A T M E N T S	NGT PLACEMENT CHECKED	☐ YES @ ☐ N/A	☐ YES @ ☐ N/A	☐ YES @ ☐ N/A
	FEEDING TUBE RESIDUAL (cc's)	☐ N/A cc's _____	☐ N/A cc's _____	☐ N/A cc's _____
	ORAL SUCTIONING	☐ YES @ ☐ N/A	☐ YES @ ☐ N/A	☐ YES @ ☐ N/A
	NASO-TRACH SUCTIONING	☐ YES @ ☐ N/A	☐ YES @ ☐ N/A	☐ YES @ ☐ N/A
	TRACH. CARE	☐ YES @ ☐ N/A	☐ YES @ ☐ N/A	☐ YES @ ☐ N/A
	FOLEY IRRIGATION	☐ YES @ ☐ N/A	☐ YES @ ☐ N/A	☐ YES @ ☐ N/A
	TRACTION	☐ YES TYPE _____ ☐ N/A	☐ YES TYPE _____ ☐ N/A	☐ YES TYPE _____ ☐ N/A
	ANTI-EMBOLIC STOCKINGS	☐ YES ☐ NO	☐ YES ☐ NO	☐ YES ☐ NO
	GUAIAC RESULT	☐ POS. ☐ Neg. _____	☐ POS. ☐ Neg. _____	☐ POS. ☐ Neg. lot# _____
	K-PAD	☐ YES LOCATION _____ ☐ N/A	☐ YES LOCATION _____ ☐ N/A	☐ YES LOCATION _____ ☐ N/A
	SUCTION	☐ YES LOCATION _____ ☐ N/A	☐ YES LOCATION _____ ☐ N/A	☐ YES LOCATION _____ ☐ N/A
I V	START/RESTART	BY	BY	BY
		TIME CATH SIZE	TIME CATH SIZE	TIME CATH SIZE
		# ATTEMPTS PUMP ☐ YES ☐ NO	# ATTEMPTS PUMP ☐ YES ☐ NO	# ATTEMPTS PUMP ☐ YES ☐ NO
		SITE	SITE	SITE
		# UNITS BLOOD	# UNITS BLOOD	# UNITS BLOOD
	TUBINGS CHANGED	☐ YES ☐ NO ☐ NA	☐ YES ☐ NO ☐ NA	☐ YES ☐ NO ☐ NA
S A F E T Y	BED CHECK	☐ YES ☐ NO ☐ N/A	☐ YES ☐ NO ☐ N/A	☐ YES ☐ NO ☐ N/A
	SIDE RAIL UP/ BED IN LOW POSITION	☐ X2 ☐ NO ☐ YES ☐ NO	☐ X2 ☐ NO ☐ YES ☐ NO	☐ X2 ☐ NO ☐ YES ☐ NO
	CALL BUTTON WITHIN REACH	☐ YES ☐ NO	☐ YES ☐ NO	☐ YES ☐ NO
	SEIZURE PRECAUTIONS	☐ N/A ☐ NO	☐ N/A ☐ NO	☐ N/A ☐ NO
	FALL HIGH RISK	☐ YES	☐ YES	☐ YES
	RESTRAINTS	☐ NO ☐ VEST ☐ WRIST ☐ ANKLE CHECK/REMOVED @ _____	☐ NO ☐ VEST ☐ WRIST ☐ ANKLE CHECK/REMOVED @ _____	☐ NO ☐ VEST ☐ WRIST ☐ ANKLE CHECK/REMOVED @ _____
	ISOLATION	☐ YES TYPE: _____ ☐ N/A	☐ YES TYPE: _____ ☐ N/A	☐ YES TYPE: _____ ☐ N/A
M I S C.	SPECIAL PREPS	☐ YES TYPE: _____ ☐ N/A	☐ YES TYPE: _____ ☐ N/A	☐ YES TYPE: _____ ☐ N/A
	SPECIMEN COLLECTED	☐ SENT TO LAB ☐ NA TYPE: _____	☐ SENT TO LAB ☐ NA TYPE: _____	☐ SENT TO LAB ☐ NA TYPE: _____
	SPECIMEN COLLECTED	☐ SENT TO LAB ☐ NA TYPE: _____	☐ SENT TO LAB ☐ NA TYPE: _____	☐ SENT TO LAB ☐ NA TYPE: _____
	PROCEDURE/DIAG. TEST			
	PHYSICIAN'S VISITS (NAME/TIME)			

(continues)

(continued)

PATIENT CARE RECORD
PATIENT ASSESSMENT

INSTRUCTIONS: CHECK □ OR FILL IN BLANKS AS APPROPRIATE

SHIFT ASSESSMENT	DAY Time _____	EVENING Time _____	NIGHT Time _____
1. NEUROLOGICAL/ LEVEL OF CONSCIOUSNESS	□ ORIENTED □ DISORIENTED □ CONSCIOUS □ UNCONSCIOUS □ ALERT □ LETHARGIC □ SEDATED □ OTHER _____ PUPILS: □ EQUAL □ UNEQUAL □ DESCRIBE	□ ORIENTED □ DISORIENTED □ CONSCIOUS □ UNCONSCIOUS □ ALERT □ LETHARGIC □ SEDATED □ OTHER _____ PUPILS: □ EQUAL □ UNEQUAL □ DESCRIBE	□ ORIENTED □ DISORIENTED □ CONSCIOUS □ UNCONSCIOUS □ ALERT □ LETHARGIC □ SEDATED □ OTHER _____ PUPILS: □ EQUAL □ UNEQUAL □ DESCRIBE
2. PAIN	□ NO □ YES □ SEE NARRATIVE	□ NO □ YES □ SEE NARRATIVE	□ NO □ YES □ SEE NARRATIVE
3. EMOTIONAL BEHAVIOR	□ COOPERATIVE □ UNCOOPERATIVE □ COMBATIVE □ CALM □ ANXIOUS □ DEPRESSED □ UPSET □ ANGRY	□ COOPERATIVE □ UNCOOPERATIVE □ COMBATIVE □ CALM □ ANXIOUS □ DEPRESSED □ UPSET □ ANGRY	□ COOPERATIVE □ UNCOOPERATIVE □ COMBATIVE □ CALM □ ANXIOUS □ DEPRESSED □ UPSET □ ANGRY
4. RESPIRATORY	□ EVEN □ UNEVEN □ SOB □ LABORED □ SHALLOW □ DEEP BREATH SOUNDS CLEAR □ L □ R RALES □ L □ R RHONCI □ L □ R WHEEZES □ L □ R CONGESTED □ L □ R O₂ L/M □ NC □ MASK □ REBREATHER	□ EVEN □ UNEVEN □ SOB □ LABORED □ SHALLOW □ DEEP BREATH SOUNDS CLEAR □ L □ R RALES □ L □ R RHONCI □ L □ R WHEEZES □ L □ R CONGESTED □ L □ R O₂ L/M □ NC □ MASK □ REBREATHER	□ EVEN □ UNEVEN □ SOB □ LABORED □ SHALLOW □ DEEP BREATH SOUNDS CLEAR □ L □ R RALES □ L □ R RHONCI □ L □ R WHEEZES □ L □ R CONGESTED □ L □ R O₂ L/M □ NC □ MASK □ REBREATHER
5. GASTRO-INTESTINAL	BOWEL SOUNDS □ NORMAL □ ABSENT □ HYPERACTIVE □ HYPOACTIVE □ HOB↑____° ABDOMINAL DISTENSION □ NO □ YES ABDO. CHARACTERISTICS □ SOFT □ FIRM □ RIGID NAUSEA: □ NO □ YES EMESIS □ NO □ YES EMESIS: #_____ , COLOR _____ STOOL: # _____ , CONSISTENCY _____ COLOR _____ NGT DRAINAGE □ NO □ YES COLOR _____ TUBE FEEDING TYPE _____ □ CONT RATE □ BOLUS CC'S @	BOWEL SOUNDS □ NORMAL □ ABSENT □ HYPERACTIVE □ HYPOACTIVE □ HOB↑____° ABDOMINAL DISTENSION □ NO □ YES ABDO. CHARACTERISTICS □ SOFT □ FIRM □ RIGID NAUSEA: □ NO □ YES EMESIS □ NO □ YES EMESIS: #_____ , COLOR _____ STOOL: # _____ , CONSISTENCY _____ COLOR _____ NGT DRAINAGE □ NO □ YES COLOR _____ TUBE FEEDING TYPE _____ □ CONT RATE □ BOLUS CC'S @	BOWEL SOUNDS □ NORMAL □ ABSENT □ HYPERACTIVE □ HYPOACTIVE □ HOB↑____° ABDOMINAL DISTENSION □ NO □ YES ABDO. CHARACTERISTICS □ SOFT □ FIRM □ RIGID NAUSEA: □ NO □ YES EMESIS □ NO □ YES EMESIS: #_____ , COLOR _____ STOOL: # _____ , CONSISTENCY _____ COLOR _____ NGT DRAINAGE □ NO □ YES COLOR _____ TUBE FEEDING TYPE _____ □ CONT RATE □ BOLUS CC'S @
6. INTEGUMENT	SKIN COLOR: □ NORMAL □ PALE □ CYANOTIC □ FLUSHED □ JAUNDICED □ MOTTLED SKIN CHARACTER: □ WARM □ COOL □ MOIST □ DRY SKIN TURGOR: EDEMA □ NO □ YES SITE _____ IV/HEPARIN LOCK/SITE _____ CENTRAL LINE DESCRIPTION: □ CLEAN □ ERYTHEMA □ EDEMA SOLUTION/RATE: _____	SKIN COLOR: □ NORMAL □ PALE □ CYANOTIC □ FLUSHED □ JAUNDICED □ MOTTLED SKIN CHARACTER: □ WARM □ COOL □ MOIST □ DRY SKIN TURGOR: EDEMA □ NO □ YES SITE _____ IV/HEPARIN LOCK/SITE _____ CENTRAL LINE DESCRIPTION: □ CLEAN □ ERYTHEMA □ EDEMA SOLUTION/RATE: _____	SKIN COLOR: □ NORMAL □ PALE □ CYANOTIC □ FLUSHED □ JAUNDICED □ MOTTLED SKIN CHARACTER: □ WARM □ COOL □ MOIST □ DRY SKIN TURGOR: EDEMA □ NO □ YES SITE _____ IV/HEPARIN LOCK/SITE _____ CENTRAL LINE DESCRIPTION: □ CLEAN □ ERYTHEMA □ EDEMA SOLUTION/RATE: _____
7. WOUND	LOCATION: _____ SIZE _____ APPEARANCE: _____ SKIN CLOSURE: _____ DRAINAGE: COLOR _____ AMT _____ DRESSING CHANGE # _____ DRAINS: TYPE SITE	LOCATION: _____ SIZE _____ APPEARANCE: _____ SKIN CLOSURE: _____ DRAINAGE: COLOR _____ AMT _____ DRESSING CHANGE # _____ DRAINS: TYPE SITE	LOCATION: _____ SIZE _____ APPEARANCE: _____ SKIN CLOSURE: _____ DRAINAGE: COLOR _____ AMT _____ DRESSING CHANGE # _____ DRAINS: TYPE SITE
8. GENITOURINARY	URINATING □ NO □ YES CLARITY _____ COLOR _____ INCONTINENT □ NO □ YES CATHETER: □ FOLEY □ STRAIGHT _____ c.c. GU IRRIGANT TYPE RATE	URINATING □ NO □ YES CLARITY _____ COLOR _____ INCONTINENT □ NO □ YES CATHETER: □ FOLEY □ STRAIGHT _____ c.c. GU IRRIGANT TYPE RATE	URINATING □ NO □ YES CLARITY _____ COLOR _____ INCONTINENT □ NO □ YES CATHETER: □ FOLEY □ STRAIGHT _____ c.c. GU IRRIGANT TYPE RATE
9. CARDIOVASCULAR	HEART: □ REGULAR □ IRREGULAR HEART SOUNDS: □ NORMAL □ ABNORMAL _____ TELEMETRY # RHYTHM	HEART: □ REGULAR □ IRREGULAR HEART SOUNDS: □ NORMAL □ ABNORMAL _____ TELEMETRY # RHYTHM	HEART: □ REGULAR □ IRREGULAR HEART SOUNDS: □ NORMAL □ ABNORMAL _____ TELEMETRY # RHYTHM
10. EXTREMITIES	□ FULL ROM ALL EXTREMITIES □ ROM DEFICITS: _____ □ RU □ LU □ RL □ LL PULSES: _____ RT. RADIAL □ NO □ YES LT. RADIAL □ NO □ YES RT. PEDALS □ NO □ YES LT. PEDALS □ NO □ YES	□ FULL ROM ALL EXTREMITIES □ ROM DEFICITS: _____ □ RU □ LU □ RL □ LL PULSES: _____ RT. RADIAL □ NO □ YES LT. RADIAL □ NO □ YES RT. PEDALS □ NO □ YES LT. PEDALS □ NO □ YES	□ FULL ROM ALL EXTREMITIES □ ROM DEFICITS: _____ □ RU □ LU □ RL □ LL PULSES: _____ RT. RADIAL □ NO □ YES LT. RADIAL □ NO □ YES RT. PEDALS □ NO □ YES LT. PEDALS □ NO □ YES
SIGNATURES AND INITIALS (ONE ONLY)	RN _____ LVN _____	RN _____ LVN _____	RN _____ LVN _____

PAGE-5

(continues)

(continued)

TIME/#	NURSING PROGRESS NOTES / PATIENT OUTCOMES (CONT'D)

**Conroe
Regional Medical Center**

Interdisciplinary Patient/Family Education Record

PATIENT/FAMILY KNOWLEDGE DEFICIT

Init.	Signature & Title	Init.	Signature & Title

A D D R E S S O G R A P H

REFERENCE CODES:

Patient Educational Need/Problem	Discipline	Learning Barriers	Learner /Person Present	Teaching Method	Evaluation of Learning
1. Medication 2. Food & Drug Interaction 3. Equipment 4. Rehabilitation Techniques 5. Tests/Procedures 6. Surgery: Pre-op / Post-op 7. Nutrition Counseling 8. Responsibilities of patients in their care 9. Available commun. resources 10. Miscellaneous	N = Nursing RD = Dietitian CM = Case Manager Rx = Pharmacy SS = Social Worker RT = Resp. Therapist ST = Speech Therapy PT = Physical Therapy OT = Occup. Therapy HB = Hyperb. Wound O = Other	1. Language 2. Memory 3. Vision 4. Hearing 5. Fatigue/ Pain 6. Emotional 7. Ability to grasp concepts 8. Access to community resources 9. Financial Concerns 10 Religious Considerations 11. Motivation 12. Cultural Factors 13. Education Needs 14. Other age-related issues 15. None	P = Patient SP = Spouse M = Mother F = Father D = Daughter S = Son F = Friend SIG = Significant Other O = Other	1. Audiovisual 2. Demo. 3. Handout 4. Discussion 5. Class/lecture 6. Translator	1. Demo. w/o assistance 2. Demo with assistance 3. Needs additional teaching 4. Verbalizes understanding 5. Needs reinforcement 6. No evidence of understanding 7. Refer to other sources

OVERALL PATIENT/FAMILY EDUCATIONAL GOAL: Upon completion of teaching intervention, patient or family demonstrates &/or verbalizes understanding of identified needs or problems.

Patient Needs Problems		Team Intervention Use number of appropriate item(s)						Comments*	Problem Resolved	
Date	Need	Disci-pline	Barrier	Learner	Method	Eval-uation	Initial		Date	Initial

* Use asterisk to indicate further documentation in Progress Notes.   ptfmrec3

(continues)

APPENDIX B-5 Interdisciplinary Record.
Reprinted with permission from Conroe Regional Medical Center Hospital, Conroe, Texas.

(continued)

REFERENCE CODES:

Patient Educational Need/Problem	Discipline	Learning Barriers	Learner /Person Present	Teaching Method	Evaluation of Learning
1. Medication 2. Food & Drug Interaction 3. Equipment 4. Rehabilitation Techniques 5. Tests/Procedures 6. Surgery: Pre-op / Post-op 7. Nutrition Counseling 8. Responsibilities of patients in their care 9. Available commun. resources 10. Miscellaneous	N = Nursing RD = Dietitian CM = Case Manager Rx = Pharmacy SS = Social Worker RT = Resp. Therapist ST = Speech Therapy PT = Physical Therapy OT = Occup. Therapy HB = Hyperb. Wound O = Other	1. Language 2. Memory 3. Vision 4. Hearing 5. Fatique/ Pain 6. Emotional 7. Ability to grasp concepts 8. Access to community resources 9. Financial Concerns 10 Religious Considerations 11. Motivation 12. Cultural Factors 13. Education Needs 14. Other age-related issues 15. None	P = Patient SP = Spouse M = Mother F = Father D = Daughter S = Son F = Friend SIG = Significant Other O = Other	1. Audiovisual 2. Demo. 3. Handout 4. Discussion 5. Class/lecture 6. Translator	1. Demo. w/o assistance 2. Demo with assistance 3. Needs additional teaching 4. Verbalizes understanding 5. Needs reinforcement 6. No evidence of understanding 7. Refer to other sources

Patient Needs Problems		Team Intervention Use number of appropriate item(s)						Comments*	Problem Resolved	
Date	Need	Disci-pline	Barrier	Learner	Method	Eval-uation	Initial		Date	Initial

* Use asterisk to indicate further documentation in Progress Notes

Glossary

KEY TERMS

Actual nursing diagnosis: a label approved by NANDA, classifying specific client problems or needs

Analyze: the process of rationalizing, questioning, and classifying information to reach a conclusion about a client's needs

Assessment: the effect of gathering data, organizing the data, and then documenting the data

Auscultation: listening for sounds within the body, usually with a stethoscope

Baseline data: information initially collected, forming the client's database, used for future comparison

Care plan: written documentation of the second and third steps of the nursing process which cites the client's problems/needs, goals/outcomes of care, and nursing interventions to treat the problems/needs

Client centered: focused on the client

Closed question: communication technique consisting of questions that can be answered briefly with yes-or-no or one-word responses

Closure: the phase of the interview in which all information has been collected and summarized

Collaboration: an act of communicating with other disciplines/parties for the purpose of decision making or problem solving

Collaborative problem: monitoring for the onset of certain physiological risk complications

Confidentiality: nondisclosure of information obtained by the health care team about a client; this information is considered privileged and cannot be disclosed to a third party without the client's consent

Critical thinking: a purposeful, deliberate method of thinking used in search for meaning

Data clustering: technique used to group related or like data; helps determine relatedness of data; provides confirmation of existing problem

Decision making: a skill used throughout the nursing process; process of applying judgments based on systematic and scientific theories

Defining characteristics: clinical criteria representing the presence of diagnostic facts; signs and symptoms indicating a specific nursing diagnosis

Dependent nursing interventions: actions requiring an order from a physician or another health care professional

Diagnosis: classification of a disease, condition, or human response determined by scientific evaluation of signs and symptoms, history, and diagnostic studies

Discharge planning: planning that requires analysis of the client's present health status and anticipates the client's needs after discharge for continued care

Discontinue: to terminate the portion of the care plan once the client has achieved the goal

Documentation: the process of recording assessment data, the client's health status, care provided, and response to care; includes written evidence of the interactions between and among health care professionals, clients and their families, and health care organizations

Etiology: cause or condition most likely to be involved in the development of a problem

Evaluation: appraisal of results through judicious reasoning; the fifth step of the nursing process

Evaluative statement: written statement identifying the client's progress toward goal achievement and problem resolution

Expected outcome: probable results; a detailed statement describing methods through which a goal will be achieved

Focus charting: a documentation method which includes written evidence of data, action, and response (DAR)

Goal: broad aim, intent, or objective

Goal attainment: achieved when the subject of the goal demonstrates the stated behavior within the specified time frame

Holistic: caring for the total person, including physical, emotional, social, spiritual, and economic needs of the client

Implementation: the fourth step of the nursing process during which nursing interventions specified in the care plan are executed

Independent nursing interventions: nursing actions initiated by the nurse, not requiring direction or an order from another health care professional

Inspection: systematic process of observation, which includes visual examination of the external surface of the body, as well as its movements and posture

Interdependent nursing interventions: nursing actions developed in collaboration or consultation with other health care professionals to gain another's viewpoint

Interpret: analyze the meaning and its significance

Interview: a communication exchange between the client and nurse

Introduction phase: the phase of an interview in which the goals of the interview are stated

JCAHO: Joint Commission on Accreditation of Healthcare Organizations: a surveying body which certifies clinical and organization performance of an institution following established guidelines

Kardex: a condensed reference tool used during change-of-shift report and as a quick reference throughout the shift; this tool includes basic client care information

Long-term goal: goal that may not be achieved prior to discharge from care, but may require continued attention, usually over weeks to months

Measurable: able to be quantified

Medical diagnosis: illness, condition, or pathological state for which treatment is directed by a licensed physician

Modification: alteration or revision of original care plan

NANDA: North American Nursing Diagnosis Association, international group responsible for the development and refinement of nursing diagnoses

Narrative charting: a documentation method, for which the nurse records complete data relating to the client as progress notes, sometimes supplementing notes with flow sheets

Nursing diagnosis: a label approved by NANDA identifying specific client problems/ needs; means of describing health problems which nurses are licensed to treat, including physical, sociological, or psychological; the process of identifying client problems and needs; recognized as the second step of the nursing process

Nursing interventions: prescriptions for specific actions to be carried out by nurses to promote, maintain, or restore health; specified activities executed by the nursing team that benefit the client in a predictable manner

Nursing process: an orderly, step-by-step, problem-solving method of providing nursing care; the five steps are assessment, diagnosis, planning, implementation, and evaluation

Objective data: what can be observed, measured, or felt by someone other than the person experiencing the phenomenon

Observation: skill of watching thoughtfully and deliberately using the senses, touch, sight, smell, and hearing

Open-ended question: interviewing technique that promotes client elaboration about a particular concern or problem

Palpation: process of examining by applying the hands or fingers to the external sur-face of the body to detect evidence of disease or abnormalities in organs

Percussion: physical examination technique that uses fingertips, cup of the hand, fist, or percussion hammer to hear sounds or feel vibrations

PIE charting: a method of documentation which includes written evidence of each problem, intervention, and evaluation

Planning: the third step of the nursing process, which includes identifying priority prob-lems and interventions, setting realistic goals and expected outcomes, determining appropriate nursing interventions and scientific rationale, determining collabora-tion needs, and communicating the proposed care plan through documentation

Prioritize: to impose an order or rank of precedence

Priority: estimated to be more important

Problem: the identified label of a client's health problem or response to the medical condition or therapy for which nursing may intervene; also known as the nursing diagnosis

Problem solving: the procedure of deliberate, thoughtful steps instituted for data col-lection, problem identification, planning for resolution, execution of interventions

Problem statement: consists of the diagnostic label (NANDA nursing diagnosis), etiology or risk factor, and defining characteristics (if stating an actual problem)

Process: a series of planned actions or operations directed toward a particular result or goal

Rationale: the underlying reason behind a specific response

Reporting: includes verbal communication of facts regarding the client's health status and care being provided

Revision: the process of rewriting, amending, or improving

Risk nursing diagnosis: diagnostic label preceded by the phrase *risk for;* determined for potential problems the client is at risk for developing, where specific risk factors are present

Short-term goal: goal that usually must be met prior to discharge or progress to a less acute level of care; goal usually met within hours or days

Social communication: casual conversation, spontaneous and with no planned agenda

Strength: area of positive functioning in the client, used to support the care plan, such as the desire to maintain a healthy diet, family support, or desire to get well

Subjective data: symptom; what the client reports, believes, or feels

Therapeutic communication: conversation which is purposeful, goal-directed, focused on the client, and planned, creating a beneficial outcome for the client

Validation: the process of ascertaining that data are factual

Verification: process of providing confirmation or proof

Wellness diagnosis: a judgment based upon a client's transition from a specific level of health to a higher level of health

Wellness nursing diagnosis: diagnostic label preceded by the phrase *potential for enhanced*, determined when a client has indicated a desire to attain a higher level of wellness in a particular area

Working phase: the phase of the interview that focuses on data collection

Bibliography

Ackley, Betty J., & Ladwig, Gail B. (1997). *Nursing diagnosis handbook: A guide to planning care* (3rd ed.). St. Louis, MO: Mosby-Year Book.

Alfaro-LeFevre, Rosalinda. (1998). *Applying nursing process: A step-by-step guide* (4th ed.). Philadelphia: J.B. Lippincott.

Alfaro-LeFevre, Rosalinda. (2002). *Applying nursing process: Promoting collaborative care* (5th ed.). Philadelphia: J.B. Lippincott.

American Nurses Association. (2004). *Nursing: Scope and standards of practice.* Washington, DC: Author.

Benner, P. (1984). *From novice to expert.* Menlo Park, CA: Addison-Wesley Publishers.

Carpenito, Lynda Juall. (1997a). *Handbook of nursing diagnosis* (7th ed.). Philadelphia: J.B. Lippincott.

Carpenito, Lynda Juall. (1997b). *Nursing diagnosis: Application to clinical practice* (7th ed.). Philadelphia: Lippincott-Raven.

DeLaune, Sue C., & Ladner, Patricia K. (1998). *Fundamentals of nursing: Standards and Practice.* New York: Thomson Delmar Learning.

DeLaune, Sue C., & Ladner, Patricia K. (2002). *Fundamentals of nursing: Standards and practice* (2nd ed.). New York: Thomson Delmar Learning.

Doenges, Marilynn E., & Moorhouse, Mary Frances. (1998). *Nurse's pocket guide: Diagnoses, interventions, and rationales* (6th ed.). Philadelphia: F.A. Davis Company.

Doenges, Marilynn E., Moorhouse, Mary F., & Geissler-Murr, Alice. (2002). *Nurse's pocket guide: Diagnoses, interventions, and rationales* (8th ed.). Philadelphia: F.A. Davis Company.

Estes, M.E.Z. (2002). *Health assessment and physical examination* (2nd ed.). New York: Thomson Delmar Learning.

Nightingale, Florence. (1969). *Notes on nursing: What it is, and what it is not.* New York: Dover.

North American Nursing Diagnosis Association. (2005). *Nursing diagnoses: Definitions & classification 2005-2006.* Philadelphia: NANDA International.

Seaback, Wanda W. (2001). *Nursing process: Concepts and application.* Clifton Park, NY: Thomson Delmar Learning.

Shaw, Michael (Ed.). (1998). *Charting made incredibly easy.* Springhouse, PA: Springhouse.

Thomas, Clayton L. (Ed.). (1993). *Taber's cyclopedic medical dictionary* (17th ed.). Philadelphia: F.A. Davis Company.

University of Iowa (n.d.). *Nursing interventions classification.* Retrieved July 28, 2004 from www.nursing.uiowa.edu.

University of Iowa (n.d.). *Nursing outcomes classification.* Retrieved July 28, 2004 from www.nursing.uiowa.edu.

Wilkinson, Judith M. (2000). *Nursing diagnosis handbook with NIC interventions and NOC outcomes* (7th ed.). Upper Saddle River, NJ: Prentice-Hall, Inc.

Index